Social Group Work
with Cardiac Patients

HAWORTH Social Work in Health Care
Gary Rosenberg and Andrew Weissman
Editors

Social Group Work with Cardiac Patients

Maurice Scott Fisher Sr., PhD

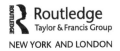

Routledge
Taylor & Francis Group

NEW YORK AND LONDON

First Published 2007 by

The Haworth Press, Inc., 10 Alice Street, Binghamton, NY 13904-1580.

Published 2017 by Routledge
711 Third Avenue, New York, NY 10017
2 Park Square, Milton Park, Abingdon, Oxon, OX14 4RN

Routledge is an imprint of the Taylor & Francis Group, an informa business

PUBLISHER'S NOTE
The development, preparation, and publication of this work has been undertaken with great care. However, the Publisher, employees, editors, and agents of The Haworth Press are not responsible for any errors contained herein or for consequences that may ensue from use of materials or information contained in this work. The Haworth Press is committed to the dissemination of ideas and information according to the highest standards of intellectual freedom and the free exchange of ideas. Statements made and opinions expressed in this publication do not necessarily reflect the views of the Publisher, Directors, management, or staff of The Haworth Press, Inc., or an endorsement by them. Identities and circumstances of individuals discussed in this book have been changed to protect confidentiality.

Library of Congress Cataloging-in-Publication Data

Fisher, Maurice Scott.
    Social group work with cardiac patients / Maurice Scott Fisher Sr.
        p. ; cm.
    Includes bibliographical references and index.
    ISBN: 978-0-7890-3100-6 (hard : alk. paper)
    ISBN: 978-0-7890-3101-3 (soft : alk. paper)
    1. Heart—Diseases—Social aspects. 2. Medical social work. 3. Heart—Diseases—Patients—Rehabilitation. I. Title.
    [DNLM: 1. Heart Diseases—psychology. 2. Psychotherapy, Group—methods. 3. Social Work—methods. WG 210 F535s 2007]
RC682.F57 2007
362.196'12—dc22

                                                                                            2007000552

CONTENTS

Foreword

For most of us, good health is something we take for granted—until it is gone. Even though we know that illness will come to each of us at some future date, we live in the shortsighted comfort of feeling well at the moment.

Of all the physical misfortunes that can befall us, few have quite the emotional impact as the discovery that something is wrong with your heart. This sad revelation can come in a variety of ways. In the case of congenital heart disease, you are born with it, a devastating blow to the parents and, eventually, a life-altering experience for the child. The heart can be affected by viral illness, by various toxins (alcohol among the most common), or by degenerative change such atherosclerosis, which can destroy the efficiency of the heart's required 100,000 beats a day.

I have always thought of the term *heart attack* as unfortunate. An attack is brought about by an enemy. Why should our most beloved organ ever attack its owner? Well, it does, and in the space of a few seconds, life can end, or be irrevocably changed.

Today much can be done to ameliorate cardiac damage. In my professional lifetime, problems that were universally fatal in years past can now be repaired, restoring normal life expectancy. Even in such cases, the person may never be quite the same: the suspicion that something is lurking in the chest that is not altogether friendly may never be far from the surface. Even if not a conscious concern, the unconscious mind may harbor memories that influence how the body operates.

The effects of cardiac illness go far beyond the individual. The family, the loved ones, the friends, the business associates may well have to adjust their relationships to the patient. Where there was once independence and strength, there may now be dependence and weakness; this makes real demands on everyone associated with the patient.

Social Group Work with Cardiac Patients
© 2007 by The Haworth Press, Inc. All rights reserved.
doi:10.1300/5739_a

In recent years, these problems have been approached through cardiac rehabilitation programs. Not only do such groups help the patient recover physically and psychologically from his or her cardiac problems, they result in a bonding with others who have had similar problems. In addition, the groups now include spouses, family, and others who are concerned with the patient's full recovery.

This is complicated business, and cardiac rehabilitation has become a subspecialty of cardiology. Much has been written to systematize teaching in patients who have survived a cardiac event. This book adds a new dimension to those studies.

Maurice S. Fisher Sr. brings a special expertise to the field. At the age of a few weeks, he was discovered to have an extremely serious congenital heart defect. Even today such a finding would bring much anxiety to the parents; in the 1960s, *terror* would have been a more fitting description. Surgical approach to a tiny baby's heart was a daunting task, being attempted in only the most serious cases as a lifesaving procedure. For more than a month after surgery, Dr. Fisher's mother sat by his oxygen tent as she held on to the shred of hope the surgeons had given her. Not only did he survive, but in adult life he has achieved much in his field of clinical social work, particularly in relation to the emotional impact of cardiac disease.

All of this gives Dr. Fisher a special understanding for the problems faced in cardiac rehabilitation. In this book, he has employed skills gained from his personal and professional experience to fashion a very readable manuscript for those interested in social group work with cardiac patients.

In my career as a cardiologist, I have had long exposure to the medical and surgical aspects of cardiac disease. It is refreshing to see the expertise of rehabilitative efforts being addressed with the same scientific intensity as interventional care. Since those days when cardiac disease was viewed as a death sentence, we have come a long way. This book is a logical step on the continuing journey to healing.

J. Hayden Hollingsworth, MD, FACC
Clinical Professor of Medicine (Cardiology), Retired
University of Health Science Center, Roanoke

Preface

The general purpose of the book is to help social workers, specifically social group workers, who provide clinical care to patients with cardiovascular disease, a more comprehensive understanding of cardiac disease, and development and refinement of skills in various areas of practice.

Chapter 1 provides an overview of the current state of cardiovascular disease from a statistical perspective relative to occurrence, incidence, mortality, relevant cardiovascular risk, and statistical cost factors. In addition, Chapter 1 deals with the connection between cardiovascular disease and the utilitarian use of social groups. Chapter 2 deals with the connection between cardiac disease and mental health issues, especially the relationship with depression, anxiety, and anger.

A patient's willingness to change his or her lifestyle in order to begin the psychosocial and physical changes for cardiac recovery include (1) the clinician clinically determining the level and intensity of his or her commitment to change, and (2) helping the cardiac patient assess his or her own level of commitment to change and cardiac recovery.

Helping the social group worker develop a better understanding of the holistic effects (i.e., heredity, lifestyle, and psychosocial variables) of cardiac disease on the patient and on the patient's family and significant others is addressed in Chapter 3. This chapter describes the linkage between social groups and the psychosocial aspects of cardiac care. Chapter 4 describes and explores the core social work groups that provide the cornerstones upon which the specialty cardiac social groups are developed.

In addition, Chapters 3 and 4 enhance the social group worker's understanding of the overall purpose, function, and structure of various groups designed to provide psychosocial help. The core group models are discussed in Chapter 3, and Chapter 4 provides a more in-

Social Group Work with Cardiac Patients
© 2007 by The Haworth Press, Inc. All rights reserved.
doi:10.1300/5739_b

depth description and discussion of these core groups upon which specialty groups are built. These groups are cognitive-behavioral groups, psychoeducational groups, skill-development groups, and interpersonal (social) groups.

Upon having a cardiac event, such as a heart attack, that is medically treated or stabilized, the treating professionals encourage the patient to change his or her life, and often these changes are related to lifestyle (e.g., quitting smoking, eating a low fat diet, etc.). However, typically, health care professionals do not assess the motivational willingness of the patient to make changes. Although motivation should be assessed on an ongoing basis, Chapter 5 describes a group work model that can be utilized to assess motivation based on the seminal work of Prochaska, Norcross, and DiClemente (1994), and suggests techniques for help to enhance motivation to change and adherence to change based on the clinical tools developed by Miller and Rollnick (1991). Furthermore, this book also addresses issues of compliance, follow-up, and a patient's follow through with his or her cardiac recovery plan. Also, methods to assess the level and degree of adherence and motivation of cardiac patients is described and discussed in Chapter 5.

Chapter 5 also serves to help the social group worker develop both a theoretical, and practical, understanding of how to match cardiac patients to appropriate groups relative to need. There are four chapters (Chapters 6 through 9) that deal with specific social groups related to specific heart events, such as heart attacks, health failure, implantable cardiac devices, and heart transplant.

Each social group underscores the use of traditional social group work methods, and relevant and current clinical interventive skills underline all of the specialty social groups discussed in this book. Each cardiac group is described and discussed in terms of the following areas:

1. *Rationale for Using the Social Group Work Model:* In this section the underlying logic for using this group model is explained.
2. *Purpose/Goals:* In this section the overarching goals are discussed and explained.

3. *Functional Characteristics:* How the group operates is discussed in this section. It includes the following aspects (e.g., a process-oriented group, a skills-development group, etc.).
4. *Structural Characteristics:* This section describes how the social group is operationally managed (e.g., whether the group is open or closed, whether the group operates homogeneous or heterogeneous relative to sex and cardiac problem).
5. *Group Leadership Skills:* This section describes and explains what instrumental social group skills are needed as well as what specific skills are needed to lead the group.
6. *Clinical Techniques Utilized:* Beyond the fundamental social group skills, this section explores the specific skills necessary and sufficient to lead the group.
7. *Expected Clinical Benefits and Outcomes from Using the Model:* This section explores positive outcomes that the social group leader strives to attain.

For each social group described, the aforementioned elements are addressed in subsequent chapters.

Specialty groups related to psychosocial issues are discussed in Chapters 10 through 13. These include social groups related to stress management, anger, substance abuse, and human sexuality among cardiac patients. These four chapters address the development of cardiac social group work outcome assessments (success versus failure in the patient being able to use specific groups to improve chances for cardiac recovery), determining skills in cardiac clinical referral when there is a need for intensive individual therapy, and cultivating the ability to assess the need for a psychiatric evaluation to determine the needs for medication such as antidepressant or mood stabilizers.

This book explores the interplay between cardiovascular illness and mental health. There are a disproportionate number of heart patients who experience depression and anxiety. Historically, anger has been related to both acute and long-term cardiac problems. Peer support among individuals dealing with a chronic cardiovascular disease is essential for recovery. Chapter 14 describes the effective use of support groups for cardiac patients.

Chapter 15 deals with issues related to coleadership. This chapter also explores the relevant positives and negatives in the use of coleadership relative to this population. Alternative ways to manage roles in coleadership are highlighted specifically related to potential barriers and obstacles. The role of a coleader in treating cardiac patients is described.

This book underscores the effects of race, age, and sex on cardiac recovery. The latest research is used to underscore clinical areas the social group worker needs to address relative to cultural awareness and sensitivity.

Finally, this book attempts to help the social group worker gain increased empathy and promote client-centered interventions to manage the psychosocial aspects of cardiac disease. This allows the social group worker to present himself or herself as a positive, honest, and authentic professional in the cardiac patient's life. Chapter 16 synthesizes the role of social group work in the psychosocial treatment of cardiac patients. Recommendations for further study are examined as well as future social group work directions are provided.

Acknowledgments

This book is the product of many hours of research, study, and reflections upon social group work practice wisdom. This effort has taken time away from the people who mean the most to me: my family. Therefore, I dedicate this book to my parents, William and Audrey Fisher, who literally stood by my side when I was an infant struggling with congenital heart disease. My parents never gave up on my cardiac recovery, irrespective of often-bleak feedback from medical professionals. Moreover, I dedicate this book to the cardiologist who was with me for more than 30 years (from grade school through college graduation and into adulthood), Dr. Hayden Hollingsworth. Dr. Hollingsworth taught me to think of my own cardiovascular problems in a holistic manner, and I gauge all the other cardiologists in my personal and professional life by his standard.

My wife, Vicky Mitchell Fisher, while enduring my time involved in this book and my often complaining, supported this work with her feedback and love. No one could have put up with me during the development of this book but Vicky.

My adult children always served to inspire, challenge, and promote my thinking. They have tolerated my involvement in this work. Scotty, Lauren, and Lee Anne have been the best to me, especially during my trials and tribulations in writing this book.

I love them all.

Social Group Work with Cardiac Patients
© 2007 by The Haworth Press, Inc. All rights reserved.
doi:10.1300/5739_c

ABOUT THE AUTHOR

Maurice Scott Fisher Sr., PhD, ACSW, LCSW, was the Mental Health Evaluator and Behavioral Health Consultant for the Virginia Transplant Center and Cardiac Rehabilitation Services at HCA/ Henrico Doctors' Hospital in Richmond for the past ten years. In his role as behavioral health consultant, he conducted five social work groups weekly and evaluated ten to fifteen cardiac patients weekly. Dr. Fisher is a licensed Clinical Social Worker, a licensed Substance Treatment Professional, a certified Substance Abuse Counselor, and a certified Sex Offender Treatment Provider. The author of numerous health care articles, he is in full-time private practice in Roanoke, Virginia. Dr. Fisher was born with a congenital heart problem and has been a life-long consumer of cardiac care.

Chapter 1

Introduction

The heart is the hardest working organ of the human body. Throughout a human being's life span, it continuously pumps blood enriched with oxygen and vital nutrients through a network of arteries to all parts of the body's tissues. In order to perform the arduous task of pumping blood to the rest of the body, the heart muscle itself needs a plentiful supply of oxygen-rich blood, which is provided through a network of coronary arteries. These arteries carry oxygen-rich blood to the heart's muscular walls (the *myocardium*). In essence, the "heart" is considered the core of one's life nurturance, existence, and ability to live.

Given the heart's significance, it's no wonder that the "heart" has become synonymous with life, love, and one's vitality and ultimate mortality. Playwrights and novelist alike have woven the concept of "heart" into myriad stories. Similarly, musicians and poets have used the "heart" as a construct representing life and health as well as love and interpersonal relationships.

In common discourse, the concept of "heart" or "having a heart" is related to one's ability to connect with others in socially accepted ways, and to having empathy for other persons' plights. Individuals often talk about being mistreated in a love relationship, or the termination of an interpersonal relationship, as feeling like a "broken heart." Generations ago, people frequently framed the death of a spouse or significant other leading to the death of the survivor as "dying of a broken heart," in the same vein as the commitment of spouses and significant others to remain steadfast in the relationship "until death we do part."

Social Group Work with Cardiac Patients
© 2007 by The Haworth Press, Inc. All rights reserved.
doi:10.1300/5739_01

1

We are simultaneously intrigued and fearful of our human heart. Generally, except for persons born with congenital cardiovascular disease (CVD), individuals do not think of, or about, their heart until a medical problem is evidenced. Nevertheless, cardiovascular problems are on the rise in America. Therefore, social group workers need to understand the overall clinical and statistical significance that cardiovascular diseases have on the patients themselves, on their respective family members, and on significant others. The effects on health care providers both directly (daily involvement of cardiac patients) and indirectly (planning for enhanced and more comprehensive psychosocial services, as well as the latent and veracious emotional transfer trauma) has to be better understood to minimize the chances of vicarious stress.

In addition, social group workers treating cardiac patients need to understand the five measurable major risk factors that negatively affect recovery: (1) high blood pressure, (2) obesity, (3) high cholesterol, (4) diabetes, and (5) the use of tobacco products along with other licit and illicit drugs. In this way, the social group worker can have a solid cardiac informational basis from which to assess, and intervene in, the treatment of specific cardiac patients as well as provide accurate information to patients who need to make informed decisions about their care.

For instance, irrespective of socioeconomic status, the prevalence of cardiovascular disease is on the increase across all races, ethnic groups, sex, and age groups at an alarming rate. Of the 70,100,000 Americans with one or more cardiovascular diseases (Centers for Disease Control [CDC] 2004, 2005a), 27,000,000 are estimated to be age of sixty- five years or older (CDC 2005a).

The following are the latest estimates of prevalence for those conditions. Unfortunately, given the often overlapping of these cardiac conditions, it is not possible to derive an aggregate number for a total. Data are from NHANES (CDC 2005a), unless otherwise noted:

- High blood pressure: 65,000,000 (defined here as systolic pressure 140 mm Hg and diastolic pressure 90 mm Hg or greater, taking antihypertensive medications, or being told at least twice by a physician or other health care professional that the individual has "high blood pressure").
- Coronary heart disease: 13,000,000

- Myocardial infarction (heart attack): 7,100,000
- Angina pectoris (chest pain): 6,400,000
- Congestive heart failure: 4,900,000
- Stroke: 5,400,000

GENERAL PREVALENCE HEART STATISTICS

Each year, heart disease is at the top of the list of the country's most serious health problems. In fact, statistics show that cardiovascular disease, or heart disease, is America's leading cause of death. At least 58.8 million people in the United States suffer from some form of heart disease. Consider the following statistics released by the American Heart Association (AHA) at the end of 1998.

One person in four suffers from some form of cardiovascular disease. These include high blood pressure (50 million people), coronary heart disease (CHD) (12 million people), angina pectoris (6 million people), myocardial infarction (7 million people), stroke (4.4 million people), rheumatic heart disease/rheumatic fever (1.8 million), congenital cardiovascular defects (1 million), and congestive heart failure (CHF) (4.6 million people) (AHA 1998).

Almost 1 out of every 2.4 deaths is from cardiovascular disease. Since 1990, cardiovascular disease has been the leading cause of death in every year except one, 1994. More than 2,600 deaths occur each day from cardiovascular disease—that is, one death every thirty-three seconds. Cardiovascular disease is the cause of more deaths than the next seven causes of death combined (AHA 1998).

It is a myth that heart disease is a "male disease." In 1996, the number of male deaths from cardiovascular disease was 453,297 (47.3 percent). In that same year, the number of female deaths from cardiovascular disease was 505,930 (52.7 percent). This is more than the next sixteen causes of deaths combined. While it is true that men generally begin suffering from heart disease at a younger age than women do, more than half of the women alive today will die from cardiovascular disease. One in three men can expect to develop cardiovascular disease before the age of sixty years. For women of the same age, the odds are one in ten. When it comes to cardiovascular events, these diseases are equal-opportunity killers, affecting both sexes, every race, and all age groups (AHA 1998).

According to the Centers for Disease Control (CDC 2005a), heart disease and stroke—the principle components of cardiovascular disease—are the first and the third leading causes of death for both men and women in the United States, accounting for nearly 40 percent of all deaths. Over 927,000 Americans die of cardiovascular disease each year, which amounts to one death every thirty-three seconds. Although these largely preventable conditions are more common among people aged sixty-five years or older, the number of sudden deaths from heart disease among people aged fifteen to thirty-four years has increased.

In 2005, the CDC reports that 696,947 people died of heart disease (51 percent of them were women), accounting for 29 percent of all U.S. deaths (CDC 2005a). The age-adjusted death rate was 241 per 100,000 populations. Heart disease is the leading cause of death for American Indians and Alaskan Natives, African Americans, Hispanics, and whites. Although cancer is the leading cause of death for Asians and Pacific Islanders, heart disease is a close second (26 percent). Heart disease death rates per 100,000 populations for the largest U.S. racial/ethnic groups are as follows: Hispanics—72; Asians and Pacific Islanders—78; American Indians—80; African Americans—206; and whites—259 (CDC 2005b).

GENERAL CARDIOVASCULAR INCIDENCE STATISTICS

Based on the National Heart, Lung, and Blood Institute's (NHLBI) Framingham Heart Study (FHS 2004; Natarajan et al. 2003), in its forty-four-year follow-up of participants and the twenty-year follow-up of their offspring, the following conclusions have been made:

The average rates of first major cardiovascular events rise from 7 per 1,000 men at ages 35 years to 44 years to 68 per 1,000 at ages 85 years to 94 years. For women, comparable rates occur ten years later in life. The gap narrows with advancing age.

Under the age of 75 years, a higher proportion of cardiovascular disease events due to coronary heart disease occur in men than in women, and a higher proportion of events due to congestive heart failure occur in women than in men.

The aging of the population will undoubtedly result in an increased incidence of chronic diseases, including coronary artery disease (CAD), heart failure, and stroke. The U.S. Census estimates that there will be 40 million Americans aged 65 years and older in 2010.

There has been a major increase in the prevalence of obesity and type 2 diabetes—the complication outcomes including hypertension, hyperlipidemia, and atherosclerotic vascular disease have also increased. An alarming increase in unattended risk factors in younger generations will continue to fuel the cardiovascular epidemics for numerous years to come. Among American Indian men of ages 45 years to 74 years, the incidence of CVD ranges from 1.5 to 2.8 percent. Among women, it ranges from 0.9 to 1.5 percent. Among American Indians of ages 65 years to 74 years, the annual rates per 1,000 population of new and recurrent heart attacks are 6.8 for men and 2.2 for women.

CARDIAC MORTALITY STATISTICS

Cardiovascular disease accounts for 38 percent of all deaths or one of 2.6 deaths in the United States in 2002. CVD mortality was nearly 60 percent of "total mortality" (CDC 2005a; Sorensent, Friis-Hasche, Haghfelt, and Beck 2005). This means that of over 2,400,000 deaths from all causes, CVD was listed as a primary or major contributing cause of about 1,400,000 death certificates. The following data highlights the rationale for Centers for Disease Control and Prevention (1993, 2004, and 2005a) labeled as the "Number 1 Killer" in the United States since 1918:

- Nearly 2,600 Americans die of CVD each day, an average of 1 death every 34 seconds. CVD claims about as many lives each year as the next five leading causes of death combined, which are cancer, chronic respiratory diseases, accidents, diabetes mellitus, influenza, and pneumonia.
- The 2002 CVD death rates were 380.4 for males and 273.4 for females.
- Over 150,000 Americans killed by CVD each year are under the age of 65 years. In 2002, 32 percent of deaths from CVD occurred prematurely (i.e., before the age of 75 years, the approximate average life expediency in that year).

- The 2002 overall death rates from CVD were 320.5. The rates were 373.8 for white males and 492.5 for black males; 265.6 for white females and 368.1 for black females.
- Based on revised 2000 population data, the average life expectancy of individuals born in the United States is now 77.3 years. According to the CDC/NCHS, if all forms of major CVDs were eliminated, life expectancy would rise to at least 7 percent (CDC 2005c).
- The CDC estimates that each year 400,000 to 460,000 individuals die of heart disease in the emergency room or before reaching the hospital, which accounts for over 60 percent of all cardiac deaths. Cardiac disease in this study included deaths from all forms of heart disease (CDC 2004, 2005a).
- In 2005, the number of premature deaths (less than 65 years of age) from cardiac diseases was greatest among American Indians or Alaska Natives (36 percent) and blacks (31.5 percent) and lowest among whites (14.7 percent). Premature death was higher for Hispanic males (24 percent) than non-Hispanic males (16.5 percent) and for males (24 percent) than females (10 percent). Hispanic whites (23.3 percent) had lower proportions than Hispanic blacks (27.5 percent) did. Non-Hispanic whites (14.4 percent) had lower proportions than had non-Hispanic blacks (31.5 percent).
- Yearly totals of out-of-hospital cardiac deaths in individuals of ages 15 years to 34 years rose from 2,719 in 1989 to 3,000 in 1996. It is quite noteworthy that although the numbers are statistically very small, the death rate increased by 30 percent in young women. Furthermore, death rates were higher among young black persons than among white persons.
- Finally, age-adjusted death rates for cardiac diseases from 1990 to 1998 declined 15 percent for non-Hispanic whites, 11 percent for non-Hispanic blacks, 17 percent for Hispanics, 14 percent for Asians or Pacific Islanders, and 8 percent for American Indians or Alaska Natives. In 1998, the rate for non-Hispanic blacks was 2.8 times the rates for Asians and Pacific Islanders (CDC 2005b).

GENERAL CARDIAC RISK FACTOR STATISTICS

Although there are multiple biologic and heritability factors that scientists are only beginning to identify and explore, there are cardiac risk factors that are tangible that need to be understood (i.e., hypertension, high blood pressure, obesity, high cholesterol, diabetes, and tobacco use and other drug use/abuse). Among adults of age 18 years older or older, the prevalence of two or more risk factors increased from 3.6 percent in 1991 to 27.9 percent in 1999. It increased significantly for both men and women and for all race, ethnic, age, and educational groups (CDC 1983, 2001, 2005b).

Among individuals with two risk factors in 1999, the most common combination was high blood pressure and high cholesterol (23.9 percent). Among those with three risk factors, the most common combination was obesity, high blood pressure, and high cholesterol (32.5 percent). Among those with four cardiac risk factors, about 43 percent had the combination of obesity, high blood pressure, high cholesterol, and use of tobacco (e.g., cigarette smoking).

Black and Mexican-American women have higher prevalence of cardiac disease risk factors than white women have, if comparable to socioeconomic status (CDC 2005b). Among the American Indians and Alaska Native of age 18 years old and older, 63.7 percent of men and 61.4 percent of women have one or more major cardiac risk factors. It is important to note that if data on physical inactivity had been factored into the analysis, the prevalence or risk factors most likely would have been much higher (CDC 2005b).

Survey data on adults aged 18 years old and older, from 1991 to 2001, showed the prevalence of reported high blood pressure, high cholesterol, diabetes, and obesity increased. Moreover, the prevalence of tobacco use remained nearly the same, and the prevalence of no known factors (or factors yet to be identified) for cardiac disease and stroke declined. Thus, it would seem that the burden cardiac diseases and stroke is expected to increase (NCCDPHP 2005).

And, finally, a study of the CDC/NCHS showed that young women and men, ages 18 to 24 years, had poor health profiles and experienced adverse changes from 1999 to 2000 (CDC 2005c). With adjustment for educational and income variables in the study, these young individuals had the highest prevalence of tobacco use (i.e., primarily via cigarette smoking). The largest increases in smoking (10 to 12 percent were among females and 9 percent among males; 34 to 36 percent of the smokers were white, while 9 percent were Hispanic women), large increases in obesity (4 to 6 percent) increase in all subgroups of individuals in the study. In addition, all groups in the study had higher levels of sedentary behavior (approximately, 20 to 30 percent) and moderate to low levels of vegetable or fruit intake on a consistent basis (35 to 50 percent). Conversely, older Hispanics and older black men (ages 65 to 74 years old) showed some positive lifestyle and behavioral changes. That is to say, the largest decrease in smoking behaviors were among Hispanic women, the largest decreases in sedentary behaviors were black men and Hispanic women, and the largest increases in intake of vegetables and fruits were also among black men and Hispanic females (CDC 2005b).

STATISTICAL COST FACTORS

The cost of CVD in 1999 was estimated at $286.5 billion—an increase of about $12 billion from the previous year. In 2005, the CDC project heart disease was estimated to cost $394 billion, including health care services, medications, and loss of productivity. In 2002, the CDC/NCHS (CDC 2005c) estimated that there were 6,813,000 inpatient cardiovascular operations and procedures performed in the United States. Of these surgical procedures, 4 million were performed on males and 2.8 million were performed on females.

In 1999, $26.3 billion in program payments were made to Medicare beneficiaries discharged from short-stay hospitals, with a principal diagnosis of cardiovascular disease. The average was $7,883 per cardiac patient discharge (Health Care Financing Review 2004). A review of the 1987 National Medicaid Expenditure Panel Survey revealed that the fifteen most costly medical conditions were ranked by health care spending. CVDs were ranked the fourth most expensive health care cost.

It is important to recognize how women are different when it comes to heart disease so that the clinical social group worker can act on those differences (CDC 2005a,b).

- *Women having a heart attack wait longer to seek care at a hospital than do men.* Women and their health care providers tend to have a false sense of security about a woman's heart attack risk. In addition, there is a difficulty in recognizing heart attack symptoms in women, since women do not always have the typical pain or pressure in the middle of the chest. The result is that it takes longer for women with heart attacks to get to the emergency room. This delay in treatment may explain why women have a higher risk of death after a heart attack.
- *Diabetes increases a woman's risk of developing heart disease more than a man's.* To date, professionals do not understand why there is this difference, but women with diabetes need to modify this risk.
- *Obesity and sedentary lifestyle are greater risk factors for women than for men.* Women should see these risk factors as stronger warning signs of future heart disease than men.
- *An African-American woman has a much higher risk of heart disease than does a white woman.* This racial difference also holds true for men, but the risk difference is greater in women, possibly because rates of diabetes and obesity are higher among African-American women.

For women, a level of HDL ("good cholesterol") below 35 is a stronger predictor of heart disease than a high level of LDL ("bad cholesterol"). Most people follow the success of cholesterol-lowering treatments by changes in LDL level. For women, it is important to pay attention to changes in the HDL level as well.

Race and ethnicity influence a patient's chance of receiving many specific procedures and treatments. Of the nine hospital procedures investigated in one study, five were significantly less common among African-American patients than among white patients; three of those five were also less common among Hispanics; and two were less common among Asian (Americans Agency for Healthcare Research and Quality 2000; National Center for Chronic Disease Prevention and Health Promotion 2001). Other studies have revealed additional disparities in patient care for various conditions and care settings including African Americans are 13 percent less likely to undergo coronary angioplasty and one-third less likely to undergo bypass surgery than are whites (Agency for Healthcare Research and Quality 2000; AHA 2005a,b).

It is important for the social group workers to be both aware of the differences between males and females, and the differences between whites versus nonwhites relative to differences in cardiovascular disease onset, course, and treatment options. In addition, social group workers need to go beyond awareness to being sensitive to these differences as they assess cardiac patients, provide clinical assessments, and determine how to tailor social groups to meet a diverse set of needs.

In a world that expects, and even demands, fairness in treatment, the course of CVD is an equal opportunity issue. That is, cardiac disease and illness knows no color, race, ethnicity, affluences, or gender in affecting people at every level and socioeconomic strata in life. But by being aware and sensitive to variations, social group workers can direct interventions in a more specific and directed fashion.

In addition, social group workers involved in the treatment of cardiac patients need to understand the level and degree of support that families from varying backgrounds need to respond to in case of chronic disease and illness. Moreover, irrespective of background, families often are divided on how they deal with a member who is chronically sick.

THE USE OF SOCIAL GROUP WORK MODELS

Social group work has a rich history of addressing an array of social and interpersonal dynamics. From its inception, social group work has successfully been utilized in myriad clinical fields of practice such as justice systems, mental health, social welfare systems (e.g., family), and health systems.

Social group work models suggested in the psychosocial treatments of cardiac patients are built upon the historic models of the Functional School (Dunlap 1996; Robinson 1930), the psychosocial model (Woods and Robinson 1996; Hamilton 1940), the problem-solving model (Turner and Jaco 1996; Perlman 1970), and the task-centered model (Reid 1992, 1996). The use of time and agency function serves to give the group a purpose and structure. The use of process and problem solving are linked to the problem-solving model and task model of social group work. And, the facilitation of individual and group-as-a-whole interaction for support and guidance is built upon the psychodynamic model of social group work.

Although the core of social groups discussed in this book are developed from the historic models, the techniques and interventive methods are derived from current group therapy models. Hence, the reader will have an inherent synthesis of both the foundations of social group work as well as those derived from the evolutionary richness of current group therapy technology.

In sum, cardiac psychosocial group work is a blend of the historic richness of social group work traditions with the current state-of-the-art group therapeutic methods in a cohesive whole in the psychosocial treatment of cardiac patients. In many instances, the social group models have been modified from the traditional intent and purpose to those that are more contemporary and relative to the state-of-the-art psychosocial treatment of cardiac patients.

The reader may use this book, either as a guide relative to best practice standards or he or she may use this book as a beginning guide in leading cardiac social work groups. In either instance, the social group worker can use this book as reference for the treatment of individuals diagnosed with CVD.

SOCIAL GROUP INTERVENTIONS CURRENTLY USED IN CARDIAC REHABILITATION

Social group work has been utilized for many years often without attention as to how effective it is in helping cardiac patients manage their disease process and their social context, such as families-of-origin, extended families, and families-of-procreation. In a research survey conducted by Lindsay and colleagues (1997), the researchers identified some of the educational and psychosocial support needs of patients undergoing cardiac surgery and their family members. They found that cardiac patients are concerned about their health and survival until the surgical procedures, as well as about the success of the medical procedures. Families in this study shared the patients' concerns, but voiced an additional concern regarding how to best support the patient during the pre- and postoperative stages. The needs identified by cardiac patients and their respective family members in this survey were found to be stable over time and within the domain of the psychosocially trained staff.

In a study evaluating the use of social groups with cardiac patients, Brown, Glazer, and Higgins (1983) reported a positive qualitative and quantitative experience with cardiac patients and their families. They noted that fear and apprehension usually accompany cardiac surgery. Experience and research have demonstrated that "many patients who have undergone open heart surgery have less than optimal psychological outcomes." This study describes the response of a university hospital to the physiological and psychological needs of the cardiovascular surgery patients during the final phase of hospitalization. To give cardiac patients and significant family members an opportunity to deal with their questions and concerns about discharge and reintegration back into their particular lifestyle, one-session education support groups were co-led by a clinical social worker and cardiovascular nurse specialist. The researchers found that reintegration back into the patient's life was significantly improved through social group involvement than for those who did not receive this intervention.

Walter, Mohan, and Dahan-Mizrahl (1992) researched the factors that enhanced the quality of life for patients after heart surgery. Their study, comprised of more than 20,000 patients, found that early identification of premorbid personalities, psychosocial counseling before and after cardiac surgical procedures, explanation of true risks, an educational program in the form of social groups in redefinition of family roles, and stressing the importance of returning to normal activities in education, employment, and society yielded improvement in all of the patients social groups, therapeutic and self-supportive. Finally, the researchers noted that general awareness of the patients' abilities facilitated an improvement in social integration and in self-reported quality of life.

In a study reported in 1991, Heitkamp and Scheib found that cardiac patients involved in both physical rehabilitation and those who had involved themselves in psychosocial group processing (thereby increasing their sense of support and connectedness), had more overall benefits in the form of high levels of physical performance.

Although the stress and anxiety experienced by patients following a heart attack are well-documented, the distress experienced by significant others when they realize that they must assume responsibility for the daily care once the initial period of hospitalization is over has been less studied. Davies (2000b) studied the effect of information provided within a social group context on overall satisfaction of help rendered as well as the effect on anxiety. The findings indicate that patients and significant others who were provided cogent information and a method for processing the information on cardiac recovery decreased both the patients' and significant others' scores on standardized anxiety and depression scales. In addition, both the cardiac patients and their significant others qualitatively expressed increased satisfaction with the predischarge information provided. The researcher notes that more qualitative, in-depth studies are needed to explore the precise needs of cardiac patients and their chief caregivers to ensure that in the future both groups are better prepared (Davies 2000a).

Asilonlu and Celik (2004) studied the effect that preoperative education provided in a social group context had on the anxiety of cardiac patients facing open heart surgery. Using a self-evaluation questionnaire for state and trait anxiety, they interviewed clients who received formal education in a social group context (the experimental group) versus those who had not received this information (control group). They found that the mean postoperative state and trait anxiety scores in the control group were slightly higher than those in the experimental group. That is, those who received help in the form of education in a social group format had lower scores than cardiac patients who had not been involved in the educational social group work process.

Stull, Starling, Hass, and Young (1999) studied the effect of assuming the role of a patient with heart failure. In this qualitative study, they found that the early phase of developing a cardiac related role was related to finding meaning in the patient's life at an early phase rather than later in the recovery process. The researchers suggested that social group work processes and interventions could positively influence the role transition among patient and their significant family members.

Previous knowledge and understanding regarding the process of recovery following surgery have been predominantly based on studies about men but now cardiac surgery becomes increasingly prevalent among women as well. In an attempt to correct this, King and Gortner (1996) studied the factors more relevant to women with cardiac problems. They found that there is a more critical desire among women to address and deal with psychosocial issues. They tended to respond to proactive psychosocial variables related to their cardiac recovery and considered them more necessary. In a study conducted by King and Jensen (1994), they explored the process that women undergo when having cardiac surgery. The researchers utilized a grounded theory approach to gain an understanding of the core process. They found that with a clearer understanding of the social process that women undergo when having cardiac surgery, health care providers will be able to participate more effectively with women through their experiences. Social groups afford people the opportunity to express their qualitative experiences in a safe, healthy fashion.

CONCLUSIONS

There is a historic precedent for the use of social group models with medical patients. In fact, the traditions of social group work had their early roots within the medical field. There is current research suggesting that social group work methods have consistently been shown as a positive change agent. In addition, the historic and current techniques of social group work have consistently been demonstrated to be a positive change agent in the psychosocial treatment of cardiac patients.

CVD does not know age, color, race, sex, gender, or age. Cardiac disease is "equal opportunity" in terms of who it affects and when. Cardiac disease is the essence of a biopsychosocial problem where one's biology/heredity propensities, social context, and psychological aspects affect the cardiac patient either prior to, during, or after the cardiac event.

Chapter 2

Correlation Between Cardiovascular Disease and Depression, Anger, and Anxiety

Of the many emotions and feelings that people experience, depression, anxiety, and anger seem to be the most debilitating and contributory in developing coronary heart diseases. Each of these emotional experiences tends to contribute to the development of heart disease and the ultimate prognosis in the treatment and recovery of cardiac patients.

DEPRESSION

Depression can affect anyone at any time. However, research over the past two decades has shown that people with heart disease are more likely to suffer from depression than are otherwise healthy people, and conversely, people with depression are at greater risk for developing heart disease (Burg and Abrams 2001). Furthermore, people with heart disease who are depressed have an increased risk of death after a heart attack compared to those who are not depressed (Frasure-Smith, Lesperance, and Talajic 1995). Depression may make it harder for administration of medications and to carry out the medical and psychosocial treatment for heart disease. Treatment for depression helps people manage both diseases, thus enhancing survival and quality of life.

Social Group Work with Cardiac Patients
© 2007 by The Haworth Press, Inc. All rights reserved.
doi:10.1300/5739_02

Heart disease affects an estimated 12.2 million American women and men and is the leading cause of death in the United States (National Heart, Lung, and Blood Institute 2002). While about 1 in 20 American adults over the age of 18 years experiences major depression in a given year, the number goes up to about 1 in 3 people who have survived a heart attack (CDC 2004; Lesperance, Frasure-Smith, Talajic 1996).

Mood disorders and anxiety disorders may affect heart rhythms, increase blood pressure, and alter blood clotting. These disorders can also lead to elevated insulin and cholesterol levels. These risk factors, with obesity, form a group of signs and symptoms that often serve as both a predictor of and a response to heart disease. Furthermore, depression or anxiety may result in chronically elevated levels of stress hormones, such as cortisol and adrenaline. As high levels of stress hormones are signaling a "fight or flight" reaction, the body's metabolism is diverted from the type of tissue repair needed in heart disease.

Despite the enormous advances in brain research in the past twenty years, depression often goes undiagnosed and untreated. Persons with heart disease, their families and friends, and even their health care professionals and cardiologists may misinterpret depression's warning signs, mistaking them for inevitable accompaniments to heart disease. Symptoms of depression may overlap with those of heart disease and other physical illnesses. However, skilled health care professionals will recognize the symptoms of depression and inquire about their duration and severity, diagnose the disorder, and suggest appropriate treatment.

Depression Facts

Depression can strike anyone. In general, depression is a serious medical condition that affects thoughts, feelings, and the ability to function in everyday life. Depression, in its many forms, can occur at any age. National Institute of Mental Health (NIMH)–sponsored studies estimate that almost 10 percent of American adults, or about 19 million people of age 18 years and older, experience some form of depression every year (NIMH 2005). Although, available therapies alleviate symptoms in over 80 percent of those treated, less than half of people diagnosed with depression get the help they need (Nemeroff, Musselman, and Evans 1998; National Center for Health Statistics 2004).

Depression results from abnormal functioning of the brain. The causes of depression are currently a matter of intense research. An interaction between genetic predisposition, life history, and experiences appear to determine a person's level of risk. Episodes of depression may be triggered by stress, difficult life events, side effects of medication, or other environmental factors. Whatever its origin, depression limits the energy needed to keep focused on treatment, especially complicated treatment instruction concerning cardiovascular problems.

Depression is common, treatable, but often unrecognized, and affects nearly 10 percent of adults, 18 years old and older, in the United States each year. Studies show that depression strikes cardiac patients at a significantly higher rate and often with devastating results (National Center for Health Statistics 2004).

Among patients with coronary heart disease, depression occurs in 18 to 20 percent of those who have not had a heart attack (myocardial infraction) and 40 to 65 percent of those with a history of heart attack (NIMH 2002, 2005; Pratt, Ford, and Crum 1996). Major depression appears to increase disability in heart patients, perhaps because it can contribute to worsening of symptoms as well as to poor adherence to cardiac treatment regimens.

In addition, heart attack survivors with major depression have three to four times greater risk of dying within six months than those who do not suffer from depression. The good news is that treating depression when it occurs in heart patients can minimize or avoid some of these serious health consequences.

Diagnosis and treatment of depression can benefit the cardiac patient through improved medical status, enhanced quality of life, a reduction in pain and disability, and improved cooperation with treatment. In addition, early treatment for depression has the added advantage of reducing the risk of relapse or recurrence of depression.

Generally, diagnosis and treatment of depression in heart patients typically goes unattended. There are myriad reasons where depressive symptoms are dismissed as the temporary low mood that is often associated with serious illness. However, in major depression, symptoms are more severe, longer lasting, and more disabling than expected. Depressive illness may also be overlooked when its symptoms are incorrectly viewed as side effects of cardiac medication. In addition, depression in an older person may be mistakenly seen as simply a part of aging. Careful evaluation can overcome these diagnostic hurdles. If co-occurring depression is present, it should be treated even in the presence of heart disease.

With treatment, up to 80 percent of all depressed people can improve, usually within weeks. Treatment usually includes medication, psychotherapy, or a combination of both. The severity of depression, the other conditions present, and the medical treatments being used must be considered to determine the appropriate treatment.

ANXIETY

Anxiety or panic attacks are one of the most common and disabling problems encountered by both mental health professionals and general medical practitioners in treating persons with heart disease. Thousands of Americans rush to hospital emergency rooms every day suspecting that they are having a heart attack, but the medical tests show that their hearts are in sound conditions (NIMH 2003; NCHS 2004).

Even after several panic attacks, a person may still believe that "unlike the last time, this [the heart attack] is for real." When a panic attack is over, patients know that their heart is normal, but during an attack, they cannot think rationally or logically. In the panic mode, catastrophic thinking replaces the normal thinking and reasoning ability. The pounding heart deafens the faint voice of the logical mind at such times. However, after ten to fifteen minutes, which is the average duration of a panic attack, a person can again believe that his or her heart is okay, but he or she would not do that during a panic attack.

The American Heart Association (1998) has noted that the body is likely to send one or more of the following warning signals of a heart attack:

- Uncomfortable pressure, fullness, squeezing, or pain in the center of the chest lasting more than a few minutes
- Pain spreading to the shoulders, neck, and arm
- Chest discomfort with lightheadedness, fainting, sweating, nausea, or shortness of breath

According to the American Psychiatric Association (APA: DSM-IV-TR 2000), a panic attack is diagnosed by the presence of at least four of the following symptoms: (1) chest pain or pressure on the chest, (2) shortness of breath, (3) dizziness or faintness, (4) sweating, (5) palpitations or accelerated heart rate, (6) nausea, (7) numbness or tingling in one or more parts of the body, (8) hot flushes or chills, and (9) the intense fear of dying, going crazy, or losing control.

It is noteworthy that the symptoms of a heart attack are similar to those of a panic attack. One may find some comfort in recent research findings that the majority of healthy people occasionally experience some type of occasional heat irregularity such as a skipped beat, pounding in the chest, or palpitation (Frasure-Smith, Lesperance, and Talajic 1995; NIMH 2003, 2006).

There is no connection between panic attacks and heart disease except that the symptoms of both are subjectively experienced similarly. Following a panic attack, some people develop intense fear about having a heart attack. They then start monitoring themselves very closely, trying to detect any signs of heart disease. Hence, when their heart rate increases, which is normal for persons under excitement, stress, or fatigue, they think they are having a heart attack. Then, the mere thought of having a heart attack sends the heart and the rest of the body into a frenzy state. Other people who do not suffer from panic attacks also experience similar cardiac changes such as heart palpitations and heart racing, but they do not get alarmed and do not view them as warning signs of an impending heart attack, stroke, or some other life threatening illness.

Researchers have noted that high levels of phobic anxiety have been associated with elevated risks of cardiac heart disease death and sudden cardiac death (SCD) among men (Budaj et al. 2005). However, until recently, no such association has been investigated among women. Researchers at Brigham and Women's Hospital and Massachusetts General Hospital, in an analysis of data from the Nurses' Health Study show that women with anxiety disorder in the form of phobic disorders, such as the fear of crowded places, going outside, or heights are at greater risk for fatal heart disease than women with fewer or no anxieties (Budaj et al. 2005). Several studies have suggested that psychosocial factors, such as emotions, anxiety, and anger are associated with an elevated risk of heart diseases, particularly death from heart disease (Mercola 2000, 2002; Rozanski, Blumenthal, and Kaplan 1999). Studies in men suggest that anxiety, specifically phobic anxiety, is related to sudden cardiac death, which occurs within one hour of the onset of symptoms and is usually associated with a lethal heart disturbance (CDC 2004; Chang et al. 2002).

The uncontrollable palpitations and quickened pulse that accompany stress and anxiety in most people are particularly bad news for those who already have cardiovascular problems. Rutledge, Linden, and Paul (2002) treated eighty patients suffering from cardiovascular disease with heart drugs amiodipine and atenolol, then made them exercise on a treadmill and took a set of psychological tests to assess their mood. During the final exercise session, 90 percent of the more highly stressed patients complained of chest pain, compared to just 40 percent of the entire group. According to Rutledge and his colleagues (2002), this finding was due to stressed heart disease sufferers being more likely to have high blood pressure than do their calmer counterparts, undercutting the impact of their medication. If they can improve their mood before starting treatment, however, they can restore their responsiveness to drug therapy. Therefore, Rutledge advises medical doctors to screen for stress and anxiety before prescribing medications, especially in patients with cardiovascular disease, so the drugs work as effectively as possible.

In another study conducted by Sherry L. Grace and associates (2004), the researchers found that over one-third of the 913 participants from twelve independent sites diagnosed with unstable angina and myocardial infarction, experienced elevated anxiety at the time of the ischemic event, and these symptoms persisted for one year in 50 percent of anxious participants. Although participants with anxiety reported more atypical cardiac symptomatology, the prevalence of typical cardiac symptoms such as chest pain did not differ based on anxiety. After the researchers controlled for the severity of the cardiac event, family income, sex, diabetes, and smoking, the following were significantly predictive of self-reported recurrent cardiac events at six months or one year: older age, family history of cardiovascular disease, greater depressive symptoms at baseline, and anxiety at six months (Grace, Hershenfield, Robertson, and Stewart 2004). In this study, only 38 percent of anxious patients were asked about such symptoms, indicating underutilization of effective psychotherapeutic treatment. In essence, beyond the effects of depressive symptoms (among other confounding variables), nonphobic anxiety appears to have a negative effect on self-reporting outcomes following an ischemic coronary event. Anxiety symptoms are underrecognized and undertreated, and examination of effects of treatment on secondary prevention must be studied further.

In addition, people who have experienced trauma stress events such as combat or urban disaster are at greater risk of developing heart disease in the future, according to new research by The New York Academy of Medicine (American Psychosomatic Society 2004). Furthermore, anxiety is often present with depression and may be one of its manifestations. Although the reverse effects of depression in patients with chronic heart failure have been well studied, the relationship between anxiety and chronic heart failure prognosis has not been addressed. In a secondary analysis of data collected for a published study of depression and prognosis in patients with chronic heart failure, Jiang and Davidson (2005) examined the relationship among anxiety, depression, and prognosis. The finding from this effort revealed that although anxiety and depression are highly correlated in patients with chronic heart failure, depression alone predicts a significantly worse prognosis for these patients.

Anxiety, which has a higher incidence in women in general, is problematic when superimposed on heart disease for a number of reasons. Higher levels of anxiety adversely affect physical functioning, interfere with role performance and role fulfillment, and increase risk for heart disease sequelae and progression. Furthermore, anxiety is a significant predictor of depression in both men and women with heart disease (Daviglus et al. 2004).

Relatively few studies have explored women's psychological or social responses to a cardiac health disruption. One study used a developmental approach to examine relationships among role experiences and anxiety in a cross-sectional study of 155 women, seven months after heart surgery (Plach and Heidrich 2002). Early middle-aged women (aged 40 years to 55 years) had more anxiety than midlife women (aged 56 years to 65 years) and elderly women (aged 66 years and older). Early middle-aged women reported a lower balance between role rewards and concerns and more incongruence between ideal and actual function than reported by their older counterparts.

Plach and Heidrich (2002) reported that midlife women (aged 38 years to 64 years) experienced greater anxiety related to problems with role performance and family responsibilities than women aged 65 years and older. Compared to men, women have higher levels of anxiety prior to a cardiac intervention (King and Gortner 1996). One year after heart surgery, women reported more anxiety, depression, and sleep disturbances than men did (NIMH 2005; AHA 1998). Women have significantly higher trait and state of anxiety throughout both the preoperative and postoperative cardiac surgery phases (AHA 1998; CDC 2005c). During the early hospitalization phase for acute myocardial infarction, women report higher anxiety levels than men (King and Gortner 1996). Even eight to nine years after a cardiac event, anxiety was significantly higher for younger women (less than 58 years) than for older women or men (King and Gortner 1996). In contrast, Duits, Duivenvoorden, and Boeke (1998), reported that during the six weeks after cardiac surgery, women had significantly fewer mood disturbances (anxiety and depression) and higher levels of satisfaction with family life than did men.

In a study comparing the anxiety experienced by age in both men and women recovering from cardiac surgery, National Institute of Mental Health (2001) noted that younger age for both men and women was a stronger predictor than gender for increased anxiety. Women's increased anxiety after a cardiac event may very well be related to changes and stressors in their social roles. They return to household tasks sooner than men, frequently as early as one week postdischarge (Hamilton and Seidman 1993), but return to paid work later than men did, if at all. Because of home and family responsibilities, women are less likely than men to enroll in cardiac rehabilitation programs, and those women who do enroll have higher dropout rates (King and Jensen 1994).

ANGER

Although depression has often been theorized as anger turned inward, there has been only a minimal support for the contrary argument, that anger is depression externalized. However, it is true that anger has been shown to have a deleterious effect on persons in general, relative to their emotional well-being, and specifically, anger has a direct and potentially deadly effect on persons already experiencing cardiac problem or have risk factors in that direction. There is an Asian saying that goes, "You will not be punished for your anger. You will be punished by your anger."

The relation of hostility to CHD and heart attacks has been debated for several decades. It was originally believed that anger was part of a personality construct called Type A, which is aggressive, extroverted, and presumed to have increased risks for heart disease. The Type A personality eventually did not turn out to be a good predictor of heart disease (Williams et al. 2000). Then, clinical interest turned toward two attributes of Type A personality: hostility and anger. The clinical evidence has increased, but is still not entirely understood. An impressive study conducted by Janice Williams and associates showed that persons who scored highest on an anger scale had almost a doubled risk of heart attack compared to those with relatively low anger scores. When the study was divided into those with normal blood pressure and those with high blood pressure, the results were surprising. Those with normal blood pressure and the highest anger scores had a threefold increased risk of heart attack. Those with elevated blood pressure and low anger scores showed no more increased risk for cardiovascular disease than those with normal blood pressure and high anger measures. It is also important to note that when controlling for race as a variable, there were no differences between blacks and whites. Those who showed moderate anger on a ten-item scale had an increased risk of heart attack or severe CHD compared to those who scored lowest on the anger scale. The authors concluded that anger-proneness as a personality trait may place persons with normal blood pressure at significant risk for coronary heart disease (Williams et al. 2000).

The deleterious effect of anger on cardiovascular health is increasingly gaining attention in the research literature. Evidence for an anger–CHD association has been derived from studies that use different measures of anger, different CHD end points, and different study designs. Trait anger, the focus of the present study, is a relatively stable personality trait that is manifested in the frequency, intensity, and duration of the anger experience. Persons with high trait anger compared to persons with low trait anger have rage and fury more often, more intensely, and with longer-lasting episodes. Persons with high trait anger, by virtue of their propensity toward anger and their long-term exposure to its pathophysiological sequelae, might be particularly susceptible to CHD. However, this association may be attenuated in persons under treatment for hypertension because many pharmacological agents used to treat this condition may reduce the expression of CHD and the physiological responses to stress.

Although anger is considered a natural and necessary human emotion, if handled in an unhealthy way, uncontrollable anger can not only damage relationships and affect professional and social growth, anger can also be a health hazard. Poor anger management can lead to premature heart disease and can cause elevations in blood pressure. In a 2002 study by Johns Hopkins Medical School, the researcher revealed that men were three times more likely to develop heart disease if they reacted to stress with anger. Evidence suggests this is because anger causes the body to release extra hormones, which constricts the blood vessels and makes the heart work harder to pump blood to the body.

Anger is no less deadly for women (Thomas 1989). A recent North Carolina study, published in the journal *Circulation,* looked at 256 men and women who had heart attacks and showed that those prone to anger were also three times more likely to have a heart attack than those least prone. Irrespective to gender, the researchers say the finding were true for individuals with normal blood pressure levels (AHA 1998; Droppleman and Witt 1993). In addition, the researchers concluded that anger could lead to heart attacks, particularly among middle-aged men and women with normal blood pressures (Deffenbacher 1995; Mercola 2000).

Having a dominant personality (one sign being a tendency to interrupt others) or a high level of irritability are two personality traits that make one prone to heart problems. Researchers have found that people who were rated as having a dominant personality had a 47 percent higher risk of heart disease in general, and those who had high scores of irritability had a 27 percent increase in heart disease risk compared to their less domineering, more easygoing counterparts (Chang et al. 2002). Also, these same researchers found that the study did not support the common belief that men display their anger and women internalize it. Thus, males and females may just express their anger differently.

Apparently, anger-induced heart problems are age blind. Researchers used the information developed during the Johns Hopkins Precursors study, first started in 1948 and continued to 1964, to see if there was a relationship between youthful anger and premature heart disease. They found that those who identified themselves as younger and had historically dealt with stress with high levels of anger were five to six times more likely to develop heart attacks before the age of 55 years. In addition, those subjects who reported high levels of anger were up to three times more likely to develop other premature manifestations of coronary vascular disease, such as angina, hardening of the arteries, higher blood pressure, congestive heart failure, and sudden death (Chang et al. 2002).

Relative to CHD, the physiology of anger is intertwined. During an outburst of anger, heart rate goes up to approximately 180 beats per minute or even higher compared to the regular heart rate average of 80 beats per minute. In addition, blood pressure goes up to 220 mm Hg/130 mm Hg or even higher compared to normal readings of 120 mm Hg/80 mm Hg. Other harmful physical and chemical changes also take place. The human body uses up sugar extremely fast, thus creating deficits. Relative to human physiology, in more primitive times, anger, aggression, and assault were one and the same. The body just knows that it is in a "fight, flight, or freeze" mode, in which it may be injured and bleeding may occur. To safeguard itself, in case of excessive bleeding, the angry person's body releases chemicals to coagulate (clot) the blood, therefore blood clots form more quickly than usual.

STATIC AND DYNAMIC CARDIOVASCULAR DISEASE FACTOR

A health risk factor is something that increases an individual's chances of developing a chronic disease. Hence, cardiac risk factors are variables that affect and increase the chances of developing heart disease. In the instance of cardiac health, a risk factor can be a personal habit (i.e., lifestyle), practice, personal attribute, characteristic, or condition that increases the overall likelihood that an individual will develop a cardiac disease or condition. Risk factors contribute to the progression of the disease or condition.

Cardiac medical and behavioral science researchers are steadily discovering more concise risk factors for cardiac disease. For example, the Framingham study has followed the lifestyles, health factors, and health records of 10,000 men and women in detail for over fifty years (Framingham Heart Study 2004).

Cardiac risk factors are typically classified as either *major risk factors,* which at least double an individual's chances of a cardiac disease or condition, or *other risk factors,* which do not, according to the most recent research data (Framingham Heart Study 2004), demonstrate a level of danger congruent with that of the major factors. Other risk factors can contribute to one's chances of developing a cardiac disease or condition in significant ways.

Another way to view cardiac risk factors is to categorize them as either *static risks factors* (factors that one cannot control or effect a change) or *dynamic risks factors* (those factors that one can influence or control). For example, one's sex, age, race, or ethnicity is static factors that are not particularly changeable. One's cholesterol, blood pressure, or uses of licit or illicit substances are within the scope of individual control, affect, or change.

The following major cardiac risk factors are typically identified as either static or dynamic:

- Increasing age (static risk factor)
- Substance use, abuse, or dependency (dynamic risk factor)
- Inactive or physically sedentary lifestyle (dynamic risk factor)
- Family history of cardiovascular disease (static risk factor)
- Gender (static risk factor)
- Elevated cholesterol (mostly a dynamic risk factor, but the latest research has revealed that the so-called "bad cholesterol [high LDL; low HDL]" can be produced by the body as well as through the foods one eats)
- Hypertension (dynamic risk factor)
- Obesity (dynamic risk factor)
- Race (static risk factor)
- Diabetes (as with cholesterol, diabetes is mostly a dynamic trait)
- Stress (dynamic risk factor)

Since cardiac patients tend to have multiple risk factors, with addition of risk factors, a synergistic effect occurs. These cardiac risk factors do not simply add up; the effects tend to multiply, making for a hazardous condition for the patient. Findings from the Framingham Heart Study (2004) suggest that cardiac patients having only one risk factor double their chances of developing either a cardiovascular disease or condition. When two or more risk factors are identified, the chances of developing cardiac maladies quadruple. When three or more cardiac risk factors are present, the probability of developing major cardiac diseases increases eight to twenty times. Unfortunately, having two or three risk factors is not uncommon. In addition, cardiac risk factors tend to occur in clusters.

CONCLUSIONS

In sum, with other conditions being equal, a person prone to depression, anxiety, anger, anger outburst, or high hostility is at a greater risk of a heart attack, or even death, than is a person with low anger or hostility. There is no question that negative emotions that are out of balance will have a profound influence on people's health. Some have suggested that more heart disease deaths result from anger than smoking and high cholesterol combined (Mercola 2000). Static and dynamic risk factors need to be considered relative to how one is affected by depression, anxiety, and/or anger.

Chapter 3

Social Group Work and Cardiac Care

INTRODUCTION

Because humans, by nature, are social and prefer social interaction, group work is a powerful therapeutic tool that is effective in dealing with the psychosocial and educational needs of persons having cardiovascular disease. The therapeutic social groups described in this book are those that have trained professional leaders and a specific intent to treat the social and psychological aspects of heart disease.

Social group work has advantages over other modes of treatment. These include positive peer support, a reduction in patients' sense of isolation, real-life examples of cardiac disease survivorship, help from peers in coping with cardiac disease as well as other ancillary social problems (e.g., depression, anxiety, and anger), information and feedback from peers, a forum to practice new family coping and adjustment skills, and social skills training related to ongoing cardiac care. In addition, social groups allow for peer confrontation that decrease denial and help to focus the patient on the realities and medical complexities of cardiac disease, as well as enhance hope, support, and encouragement necessary to embrace cardiac recovery.

In a 1992 survey (Dies 1992b), the American Group Psychotherapy Association divided group therapists into three categories according to their orientation in leading groups—psychodynamic, interpersonal, or action-oriented. The psychodynamic orientation seeks cognitive change that is intrapsychic, and thereby, positively affects the patients' schemata, or how they perceive the world. The interpersonal approaches

Social Group Work with Cardiac Patients
© 2007 by The Haworth Press, Inc. All rights reserved.
doi:10.1300/5739_03

focus primarily on the personal interactions and relationships among the group members, as typified by Yalom's classic text (1995). Action-oriented approaches include cognitive/behavioral, Gestalt, Transactional Analysis (TA), and psychodrama—the common element being a commitment to action in addition to self-exploration. This includes not only action on the part of group members (e.g., behavioral experimentation or role-playing), but also an active leadership stance from the group therapist that may include suggestions, questions, and structured activities in addition to interpretations. The specialty cardiac social groups explored in this book will be described based on the following core social group models.

BASIC SOCIAL GROUPS FOR USE IN PSYCHOSOCIAL TREATMENT OF CARDIAC PATIENTS

Although specific group models will be explored and discussed in later chapters, there are four basic group models suggested for use in the treatment of the psychosocial aspects of cardiovascular disease. These groups represent the core of social groups needed to effectively treat the psychosocial cardiac patients.

Cognitive-Behavioral Groups

These groups allow patients to actively develop skills in identification of feelings and stressors, and helps patients to detect and challenge irrational and/or illogical thoughts and perceptions that tend to underlie typical mental health disorders such as depression, anxiety, and anger. In addition, this model helps patients to develop advanced skills in reframing negative thoughts and restructuring negative perceptions and outcome expectations (e.g., negative or faulty expectations relative to the outcome of CVD). This type of group is action-oriented.

Psychoeducational Groups

These groups afford cardiac patients the needed information to help them change their lifestyle. Social groups that provide information relative to nutrition (e.g., developing "heart smart" eating habits), stress management, and medication management are helpful for the patient in cardiac recovery. This group model is an informed blend of action-oriented, psychodynamic, and interpersonal.

Skill Development Groups

These groups are helpful in the development of proper skills that enhance cardiac functioning and output, and anger management skills in self-control methods. This group model is action-oriented.

Interpersonal (Social) Groups

These groups allow the cardiac patients who are beginning their recovery to develop healthy interactions with significant people in their lives. These groups help cardiac patients develop skills in setting healthy limits and boundaries for themselves with family, friends, co-workers, and work supervisors. This group model is interpersonal.

There are several other specialized types of social groups that do not fit neatly into the four-model classification, which nonetheless are common in psychosocial treatment of cardiac patients. They are designed specifically to help cardiac patients develop support relative to their specific cardiovascular illness from patients with similar issues, allow patients to develop connections with other cardiac patients in general, and afford cardiac patients' families the needed support, as well as those that deal more directly with specific cardiac issues unique to specific patients.

SOCIAL GROUP DEVELOPMENT
AND PHASE-SPECIFIC TASKS

Social group membership may be fixed, with a relatively small number of patients (e.g., social skills development, anger management, self-control methods). Alternatively, social group membership may evolve, with new members entering a group when they are ready for the service it provides (e.g., interpersonal social groups, and support groups). Either type of group can be ongoing and have a definite time, or the social groups can be time-limited.

The initial phase of social group development for cardiac patients is advanced by the social group worker meeting individually with each prospective group member to begin the process of developing a therapeutic alliance and to determine the level of motivation to deal with cardiac recovery. During this phase, the focus is also on forming a therapeutic alliance; reaching consensus on what needs to be accomplished within the social group context; educating each member about the purpose, structure, and function of the social group, allaying anxiety related to joining a social group; and explaining the fundamental principles of the social group context. In social pregroup work interviews, it is important to be sensitive to people who differ significantly from the group-as-a-whole whether by sex, age, ethnicity, or race, specific cardiac disorders, and so forth. Most importantly, the social group leader needs to assure cardiac patients that a difference is not a deficit and can be a source of strength for the group-as-a-whole.

Selection of potential cardiac group members is based on the patient's fit with a particular social group modality. Considerations include the patient's:

1. Proximal level of interpersonal functioning, including impulse control
2. Motivation to change lifestyle related to the specific CVD
3. Potential stability of social group involvement
4. Level and stage of recovery
5. Expectation of prosocial cardiac recovery

The first few sessions of patients' social group involvement are particularly vulnerable to discontinuation of both medical and psychosocial treatment. Overall retention rates in a social group are enhanced by patients' preparation, maximal patient involvement, feedback and negative critique, prompts to encourage attendance, and the access to wraparound comprehensive medical and psychosocial information. Timing and duration of social groups also affect retention.

Although social group workers have myriad responsibilities in preparing cardiac patients for involvement and participation in group treatments, patients also have obligations as well. A social group agreement establishes the expectations that group members have of one another, the social group leader, and the social group itself. The social group contract specifies the circumstances under which cardiac patients may be accepted or barred from the group and explains the policies regarding confidentiality, physical contact, membership outside the group-as-a-whole, social group participation, financial responsibility, and termination.

The core tasks in the beginning phase of a social group include introductions (i.e., the physical and emotional "price" of being a cardiac patient; review of the group norms, purpose, function, and structure; review of the social group agreement; and focus and direct the social group toward its work and goals). In the middle phase, cardiac patients interact, rethink their behaviors and expectations, and move toward prosocial and productive cardiac lifestyle change. The end phase concentrates on reaching closure, as well as synthesizing what has been therapeutically gained within the social group.

STAGES OF SOCIAL GROUP TREATMENT

As cardiac patients move through different stages of recovery, treatment must move with them. That is to say, therapeutic strategies and social group work leadership roles will change with the treatment of the patient.

In the initial phase of treatment, cardiac patients tend to exhibit ambivalence about managing their cardiac illness, rigidity in thought relevant to cardiac change and recovery, and constricted ability to solve interpersonal problems. Typically, resistance is a challenge to the social group worker during this time. In addition, the social group worker will have to deal with fairly solid defense mechanisms such as intellectualization, rationalization, and denial. Social groups are particularly effective in the initial phase of treatment since the typical cardiovascular patient is overwhelmed, and at times, confused and ambivalent about the disease, its treatment, course, and outcome. Information from peers in the social group is more easily accepted than from the social group worker alone.

During the middle phase of treatment, persons with cardiac disease remain vulnerable. The social group worker draws attention to positive developments, points out how far cardiac patients have progressed, and affirms the possibility of increased connection and alternative sources of satisfaction.

In the latter phase of social group work treatment, cardiac patients are typically stable enough to address situations that involve conflict, deep emotionality, and prosocial, informed decision making and judgment. A process-oriented social group may become appropriate for some cardiac patients who are finally able to confront painful physical and emotional realities. Other cardiac patients may need social groups to help them build healthier interpersonal relationships with family members and peers, communicate needs via direct communications, and develop and refine prosocial problem-solving methods.

SOCIAL GROUP WORKER LEADERSHIP, TECHNIQUES, AND CONCEPTS

Responsive and effective social group leadership with cardiac patients requires a constellation of specific personal attributes and professional practice interventions. The personal attributes necessary are: constancy in leadership, active listening, a firm identity and sense of self, confidence and expertise, spontaneity, probity, trust, and empathy coupled with a sense of humor.

Social group workers treating cardiac patients need to model appropriate social group boundaries and behaviors; resolve ethical issues; adjust their professional styles to the particular and specific needs of the social group; work only within the modalities in which they are trained; prevent the development of rigid roles in the group-as-a-whole; manage emotional contagion; motivate patients in the psychosocial aspects of cardiac recovery; avoid acting in different roles inside and outside of the group (i.e., minimize dual relationships with the patients); maintain a safe therapeutic setting (which often involves deflecting defensive behaviors without shaming the patient relative to his or her historic lifestyle and genetic predispositions; protecting the physical boundaries according to the social group purpose, structure, and function); ensure the emotional safety of the group for all participants; stimulate prosocial and direct communication among the social group members; and monitor and curtail negative emotions when it becomes too intense for the specific social group members, and the group-as-a-whole, to manage and tolerate.

Key concepts and techniques used in social group work for cardiac patients follow. Social group interventions are any actions by the group leader to intentionally affect the process of the group-as-a-whole. Interventions may be used to clarify understanding, redirect emotional energy, or halt a damaging sequence of interpersonal interactions. Effective social group workers do not overdo interventions; otherwise it would result in a leader-centered social group, which is undesirable because in social groups, the recovery process of cardiac patients emerges from the connections forged between and among group members.

Diversity plays a crucial role in social group work. It may affect critical aspects of the process, such as, what cardiac patients expect of the group worker and how patients may interpret other patients' behaviors. Social group workers should be open to learning about other belief and value systems, they should not assume that each social group member from a specific social group shares the same characteristics, and should avoid appearing as if the social group worker is trying to persuade patients to renounce their cultural characteristics. Persons diagnosed with a cardiovascular illness have other complex social and psychological issues. For many cardiac patients, social groups may be one aspect of a larger clinical concern that marshals biopsychosocial, emotional, and spiritual interventions to address important life decisions and restore faith or belief in some force beyond the specific individual.

Integrated psychosocial cardiac care from diverse sources requires cooperation with other professional members of the health care team. For example, it is imperative that all health care members working with cardiac patients with multiple diagnoses know what medications patients are taking and the rationale for prescribing the medication.

Two aspects of social group work management relates to conflict and subgrouping among members. Properly managed and directed, conflict can promote learning about respect of fellow members' differing points of view, management of emotional aspects, and negotiation and compromise within the group-as-a-whole. A central aspect of the social group workers role is as a conflict manager to reveal covert conflicts and expose repetitive and predictable arguments. The social group worker also reveals overt and covert subgroups and intervenes to reconfigure negative subgroups that serve to threaten the social group's progress.

Various types of disruptive behaviors may require the social group worker's attention. Such problems include patients who monopolize the content and/or process of the social group, who are disruptive and tend to interrupt the group, who cannot tolerate the social group and have to leave the session, who arrive late or skip sessions, who decline to involve themselves or participate in a meaningful fashion, or patients who address the problems of fellow group members and ignore their own. In addition, the social group worker should have the skills and abilities to handle various people with psychosocial emergencies or people who are anxious about disclosing personal information. The four basic cardiac social groups are described in the following sections.

RATIONALE FOR USING SOCIAL GROUP MODELS WITH CARDIAC PATIENTS

For clients who have been diagnosed with a cardiac problem, recovery can be aided by improving their social skills and the quality of their interpersonal relationships. Because social group work focuses explicitly on these issues, it is an important component of cardiac psychosocial care. Social group work authorities in the field of health care (Getzel 2004; Yalom 1995) advocate for social groups for the following reasons:

1. Groups reduce the sense of isolation, depression, anxiety, and anger often experienced by people diagnosed with CVD, who may experience a sense of relief to discover that others are struggling with similar concerns and issues.
2. Groups help install hope in persons suffering from cardiac problems such that they can experience psychosocial and biologic recovery; this generally occurs when they observe other group members who are involved in cardiac recovery.
3. Groups provide an opportunity for the members to learn how to cope with cardiac problems and enhance their understanding of their illness and its course, as well as other ancillary psychosocial problems, by observing how others with similar sorts of cardiac issues cope with them.
4. Groups can provide a good deal of new information to members through material preened by the group leader or via guest facilitators, instructors, and fellow members.

5. Groups help members to develop enhanced self-concepts (e.g., self-worth and self-image) or to modify distorted self-concepts because of the feedback and negative critique members receive from other members as to worth, skills, and abilities.
6. Groups provide reparative family experiences as the group members offer each member support and nurturance that may be lacking in their own families. Also, group interactions may help members to experiment with alternative ways to create improved interactions in their own family-of-origin and family-of-procreation.
7. Groups provide emotional and affective support when members undertake anxiety-provoking or difficult tasks in their life situation outside the group. This may take the form of encouragement, reinforcement, or coaching.
8. Groups help members to acquire the social skills they need to cope with life situations through positive, proactive means to overcome feelings of inadequacy in these situations. Groups offer many opportunities to learn social skills through observing others and being coached by other members. Group members can then try the skills out in a safe and supportive environment.
9. Group members may confront each other in very powerful ways regarding healthy alternative ways to manage the psychosocial aspects of heart disease or any other dysfunctional behaviors, which are inimical to cardiac recovery. The use of confrontation is frequently found in groups to help challenge defense mechanism and improve overall coping. The appropriate uses of confrontation must be carefully assessed in terms of the needs and capacities of the members being confronted.
10. In view of the large numbers of people who require cardiac psychosocial help, group services may create some economic advantages in the use of professional staff because of the ability of groups to help a number of people concurrently.
11. The efforts of the group treatments may extend beyond the boundaries of the group context or individual meeting by encouraging members to provide support to one another outside the group session.

CONCLUSIONS

People who develop cardiovascular disorders vary greatly in race, ethnic, religious preference, sex; thus making it an equal opportunity issue. And, unless a person is born with congenital heart problems, one does not tend to give much thought to his or her heart until a cardiac issue arises. Once one has developed a cardiac event, even those with healthy intact defenses and social coping skills will be tested. Challenges to one's social skills and adaptive skills, as well as feelings of isolation, depression, anxiety, and anger, may occur.

Traditional social group work has its roots in the medical system. The historic core aspects of social group work are relevant for the use of more specialized social group models. In addition, a sense of powerlessness, feelings of losing control, and dependency on others often accompany cardiac problems. Finally, after the initial cardiac precipitating event is stabilized, medical profession almost immediately advise patients to make change in their lifestyle (e.g., nutritional practices, develop exercises that enhance cardiac functioning, and develop healthy medication management practices). Based on the patient's stage of change seeking, need, and an assessment of the patient's typical psychosocial functioning, it is recommended to assign cardiac patients to social groups that focus on motivational modalities prior to active group therapy in more change-oriented groups (Prochaska and DiClemente 1992).

Chapter 4

Core Cardiac Social Work Group

INTRODUCTION

This chapter deals with the descriptions of the four core groups that are the basis upon which specialty groups for cardiac social groups are developed. These groups include the following: cognitive-behavioral groups, psychoeducational groups, skill development groups, and interpersonal (social) groups. These groups are fundamental in social group work treatment and intervention for patients having cardiovascular disease. As one masters these core social group protocols, the social group worker can develop specialty social groups that target specific topical areas such as the treatment of patients having had a heart attack to helping patients develop skills in stress management or anger management.

COGNITIVE-BEHAVIORAL CARDIAC GROUP THERAPY

Cognitive-behavioral therapy is a psychotherapeutic approach that is used by clinical social workers and therapists to help promote positive change in individuals, to help alleviate emotional distress, and to address myriad psycho/social/behavioral issues. Cognitive-behavioral therapists identify and treat difficulties arising from an individual's irrational thinking, misperceptions, dysfunctional thoughts, and faulty learning. Problems such as anxiety, depression, anger, guilt, low self-esteem, adjustment difficulties, sleep disturbance, and post-traumatic stress can be addressed.

Social Group Work with Cardiac Patients
© 2007 by The Haworth Press, Inc. All rights reserved.
doi:10.1300/5739_04

Many cardiac patients experience depression, anxiety, anger, or fear, as well as residual stress (Droppleman and Witt 1993; LeDoux 1998; Lesperance, Frasure-Smith, and Talajic 1996). If an individual has biopsychosocial or biologic markers toward depression, anxiety, and anger, the stress of dealing with cardiac disease will enhance these tendencies. If one does not have these leanings, the process of dealing with a major illness, such as cardiovascular disease, most likely will stimulate residual depression, anxiety, and/or anger.

Cognitive-behavioral therapy is a type of psychotherapy based around the concept that changing the way a person thinks also changes his or her behaviors and the way he or she feels. Multiple randomized control group studies have supported the effectiveness of cognitive-behavioral therapy for treating depression and anxiety (Beck and Emery 1985; Beck, Rush, Shaw, and Emery 1979). More specifically, there is substantial evidence that cognitive-behavioral therapy is significantly more effective than no treatment at all.

There is consistent and growing clinical evidence that cognitive-behavioral techniques can help patients manage their depression, anxiety, and anger in more healthy, prosocial, and proactive ways.

Rationale for Using the Cognitive-Behavioral Group Work Model

The general rationale for involving cardiac patients in a cognitive-behavioral social group is that there are many cardiac patients who have gross difficulty in managing their mood. Since one's mood, or feelings, cannot be changed in isolation, the use of a cognitive-behavioral group helps patients develop skills in changing their thought, perceptions, and cognitive schemas (an individual's worldview) that promote negative feelings and enhances stress.

Oftentimes, patients enter into cardiac care feeling fearful, depressed, and anxious. Their feelings are intense. Since one cannot simply change these feelings, the cardiac patient needs to develop and refine skills in identifying feelings, both positive and negative, detecting underlying negative thoughts, perceptions, and schemata, as well as actively challenge negative thoughts, reframe negative perceptions, and restructure negative schemata.

Irrespective of whether depression, anxiety, or anger occurred prior to the cardiac event, or occurred during or after the cardiac event, these emotions need to be addressed to maximize the patient's cardiac recovery both physically as well as emotionally. In assessing cardiac patients prior to psychosocial group treatment, the clinician may find that there is a family-of-origin or extended family history of depression, anxiety, or anger management difficulties. These premorbid clinical findings are considered endogenous. On the other hand, the clinician may find that there is no family or personal history of these mental health maladies, but they emerge secondary to the cardiac event. These postmorbid clinical findings are considered exogenous. Either way, these mental health issues need to be systematically dealt with in ways that promote self-control. In some cases, the cardiac patient may need to be referred for a psychiatric evaluation to rule out the need for a medication intervention (i.e., antidepressant, antianxiety, or mood stabilizing medications).

Purpose or Goals

The overarching purpose of having cardiac patients to participate in a cognitive-behavioral social group is to develop specific skills in mood (e.g., depression, anxiety, and anger) and stress management, so that they can control their moods/feelings and make informed decisions based on emotional reaction.

Cognitive-behavioral therapy is a form of psychotherapy that emphasizes the role of rational thinking in how individuals feel and behave. A central tenet of this approach is that an individual's thoughts, not outside people or events, cause feelings and behaviors. When individuals experience unwanted feelings and behaviors, cognitive-behavior therapists identify the root of these feelings and behaviors and endeavor to change the way the individual thinks in order to replace this thinking with thoughts that lead to more desirable reactions (Pucci 2005). Cognitive therapy is essentially a method that identifies thoughts that produce negative or painful feelings, as well as result in maladaptive behavior or reactions. Beck (1995) discovered that the primary point of intervention was at the level of a person's thoughts, and that if changes are made in thinking (automatic thoughts, assumptions, and core beliefs), changes in emotions and behavior will follow. Furthermore, behavioral techniques and strategies are employed, as needed, to enhance the treatment outcome (i.e., anger management, relaxation training, graduated exposure to feared situations, assertiveness training). The course of treatment is typically brief, and people usually experience relatively rapid relief and enduring progress.

Cognitive therapy's elegantly simple model has proven to be the most powerful and effective type of psychological treatment in outcome studies conducted over the past several decades. Due to the availability of literature and training of professionals in cognitive-behavioral therapy, this model currently enjoys widespread popularity and is practiced by many qualified professionals throughout the United States and internationally.

Functional Characteristics

Typically, cognitive-behavioral social groups serve the role of skill development and are conducted in a finite number of sessions. The cognitive-behavioral social group focuses on developing skills in the following areas:

- Understanding of the critical triangle wherein cognitions (thoughts) and actions (behaviors) influence moods
- Challenging irrational beliefs, thoughts, and perceptions as well as more fixed cognitive schemas that are a product of how individuals are socialized and subsequently see the world in which they live
- Relaxation education and training
- Self-monitoring of negative thoughts and perceptions
- Cognitive rehearsal or role-play, whereby patients can practice skills in vivo
- Thought stopping, or thought blocking—this is where patients can develop skills in immediately changing their thoughts without a need to process the antecedents
- Communication skills training
- Assertiveness skills training
- Social skills training
- Bibliotherapy—this is where patients can use literature to supplement their group experiences
- Homework assignments—this gives the social group worker an opportunity to administer self-assessment instruments and assess how well the patients have inculcated the basic principles of cognitive-behavioral techniques

Structural Characteristics

The structure of this proposed group is typically time-limited and skill-focused. The cognitive-behavioral social group should be ongoing, close-ended, relative to accepting new members to enhance session consistency. The group can be either homogeneous or heterogeneous in relation to gender, cardiac disease type, and/or the psychosocial functioning of the prospective members.

Group Leadership Skills

The social group worker facilitating a cognitive-behavioral model for cardiac patients needs fairly advanced skills in the use of cognitive-behavioral skill development. Also, the social group worker needs to have a good working knowledge in the appropriate use of relaxation skills development, communication skills, and assertiveness skills development. The social group worker also needs to have a working knowledge of Choice Theory (Glasser 1998), that is, in any given situation, such as making an informed decision about one's health care, there are multiple choices. Unfortunately, one does not have the opportunity to control the outcome of any one choice since there are myriad potential outcomes. For example, one can choose, based on the best medical input, to have a bypass operation out of clinical recommendations, but this choice comes with myriad risks and outcomes over which the cardiac patient has no control (e.g., a successful outcome, medical complication, or even death).

Clinical Techniques Utilized

Given that many cardiac patients enter into treatment with fixed thoughts and perceptions concerning the outcome of cardiovascular disease, it is suggested that a specific form of cognitive-behavioral social group therapy be used.

Schema-focused cognitive therapy is the approach developed by Jeffrey E. Young, a protégée of Dr. Beck. Young and his colleagues (Young, Weishaar, and Klosko 2003) found a significant segment of people who came for treatment, but had perplexing difficulty in benefiting from the standard approach. He discovered that these people typically had long-standing patterns or themes in thinking and feeling—and consequently in behaving or coping—that required different means of intervention. Young's attention turned to methods of helping patients to address and modify these deeper patterns or themes, also known as "schemas" or "lifetraps." The *schemas* that are targeted in treatment are enduring and self-defeating patterns that typically begin early in life, get repeated and elaborated upon, cause negative/dysfunctional thoughts and feelings, and pose obstacles for accomplishing one's goals and meeting one's needs. Although schemas are usually developed early in one's life (i.e., during childhood or adolescence), they can also form later in adulthood. These schemas are perpetuated behaviorally through the coping styles of schema maintenance, schema avoidance, and schema compensation. Young's model centers on helping the person to break these patterns of thinking, feeling, and behaving, which are often very tenacious (Young 2003; Young, Weishaar, and Klosko 1999).

In formulating the schema-focused approach, Young combined the best aspects of cognitive-behavioral, experiential, interpersonal, and psychoanalytic therapies into one unified model of treatment. Through Young's work and the efforts of those trained by him, schema-focused therapy has shown remarkable results in helping people to change patterns, which they have lived with for a long time, even when other methods and efforts they have tried before have been largely unsuccessful (Young, Weishaar, and Klosko 1999).

Some of the common schemas assessed in clinical settings are as following:

- *Emotional deprivation:* The belief and expectation that one's primary needs will never be met and the sense that no one will nurture, care for, guide, protect, or empathize with the patient.
- *Abandonment:* The belief and expectation that others will leave, others are unreliable, relationships are fragile, loss is inevitable, and that you will ultimately wind up alone.
- *Mistrust/abuse:* The belief that others are abusive, manipulative, selfish, or looking to hurt or use an individual. Others are not to be trusted.
- *Defectiveness:* The belief that you are flawed, damaged, or unlovable and you will thereby be rejected.
- *Social isolation:* The pervasive sense of aloneness, coupled with a feeling of alienation.

- *Vulnerability:* The sense that the world is a dangerous place, that disaster can happen at any time, and that an individual will be overwhelmed by the challenges that lie ahead.
- *Dependence/incompetence:* The belief that one is unable to effectively make his or her own decisions, that one's judgment is questionable and that a person needs to rely on others to help get through day-to-day responsibilities.
- *Enmeshment/undeveloped self:* The sense that an individual does not have an identity or "individuated self" that is separate from one or more significant others.
- *Failure:* It is the expectation that one will fail or belief that a person cannot perform well enough.
- *Subjugation:* It is the belief that one must submit to the control of others, or else punishment or rejection will be forthcoming.
- *Self-sacrifice:* The belief that one should voluntarily give up of one's own needs for the sake of others, usually to a point that is excessive.
- *Approval-seeking/recognition-seeking:* It is the sense that approval, attention, and recognition are far more important than genuine self-expression and being true to oneself.
- *Emotional inhibition:* The belief that one must control his or her self-expression or others will reject or criticize the person.
- *Negativity/pessimism:* It is the pervasive belief that the negative aspects of life outweigh the positive, along with negative expectations for the future.
- *Unrelenting standards:* The belief that you need to be the best, always striving for perfection or to avoid mistakes.
- *Punitiveness:* It is the belief that people should be harshly punished for their mistakes or shortcomings.
- *Entitlement/grandiosity:* The sense that one is special or more important than others are, and that one does not have to follow the rules like other people even though it may have a negative effect on others. Also, this can manifest itself in an exaggerated focus on superiority for the purpose of having power or control.
- *Insufficient self-control/self-discipline:* It is the sense that one cannot accomplish one's goals, especially if the process contains boring, repetitive, or frustrating aspects. Also, that a person cannot resist acting on impulses, which leads to detrimental results.

In addition, the social group worker should have a good working knowledge of helping individuals: (1) identify negative behaviors and stress; (2) detect underlying negative thoughts, perceptions, and schemas; and (3) actively challenge and reframe negative thoughts and perceptions as well as restructure negative schemas that contribute to depression, anxiety, and depression.

Expected Clinical Benefits and Outcomes

One of the key outcomes expected is that the client will be able to understand the reciprocal interactive relation between thoughts and perceptions, behaviors and feelings (i.e., affective response); a change in thoughts (perceptions and schemas) that directly influences one's mood (feelings); that an individual's behaviors (action) also affects one's mood; and that they cannot simply change their moods (feelings) without either a change in cognitions or behaviors. The cardiac patient cannot simply change his or her mood, which is nothing more or less than an emotional reading of where the client is at a particular point in time. Simply put, one cannot simply change his or her mood without either changing one's thoughts or behaviors. From a cognitive-behavioral perspective, it is noteworthy that although one cannot control what thoughts are stimulated by the environment, individuals can learn to manage what thoughts one desires to keep versus those one does not want to keep.

Cardiac patients also learn what most promotes interpersonal conflict, stress, and distresses are cognitive schemas and perceptions. Schemas are the way in which an individual sees and interacts in the world. Typical cognitive schemas are developed through socialization either from the family-of-origin, significant others (e.g., teachers, clergy), or through other social institutions (i.e., high school, college, military involvements).

Individual perceptions develop by interacting in the social context in which individuals live and interact. Perceptions are not real, but are one's cognitive and conceptual understanding as to what is real. For example, some see the glass of water as half full, others see the glass as half empty, and others see a glass that is too big. Hence, how a cardiac patient perceives his or her world situation, and specifically the specific CVD, will directly influence how he or she will approach cardiac care and medical follow-up.

Use of cognitive-behavioral techniques is also quite useful in assessing the core of informed consent for treatment. For example, if one has a jaded view of health care or the medical profession in general, one may well deal with informed consent about cardiac procedures in a similar vein. One the other hand, if one has a positive perception of the health care system and the professionals working in this field, the cardiac patient may be more open and free to exercise free-will and self-determination.

PSYCHOEDUCATIONAL GROUPS

Psychoeducational groups are designed to educate cardiac patients about CVD in general, about specific information unique to the individual patients, and about ancillary aspects of psychosocial and health care issues. This type of social work group presents structured, group-specific content, often using prepared teaching materials (e.g., lectures), videotapes, and/or audiocassettes. Experienced social group workers will facilitate integration of presented material by helping to process information as to its applicability in members' particular situations (Maxmen 1978). In essence, psychoeducational groups provide information designed to have a direct application to the cardiac patients' lives, such as instillation of self-awareness, suggesting options for growth and change, methods on how to change the patients' lifestyle and developing an understanding of cardiac recovery. In addition, psychoeducational groups help empower cardiac patients to be active and prosocial consumers on their own behalf. Finally, while psychoeducational groups with cardiac patients may inform members about social and psychological issues influencing cardiac recovery, these groups do not aim at intrapsychic change (McLennan, Anderson, and Pain 1996). However, such intrapsychic change may occur as a latent function as changes in thinking, perceptions, and outcome expectations occur.

Cardiac topical areas that can be addressed by using a psychoeducational social group include basic cardiac anatomy, nutrition (i.e., "heart-smart" diets that include low fat foods), and medication compliance.

Rationale for Using the Psychoeducational
Group Work Model

Typically, unless one develops health problems, people generally do not think of their hearts, or about breathing. Therefore, individuals diagnosed with CVD are often overwhelmed by the multitude of changes being asked of them, as well as being overwhelmed about the cardiac disease process itself. After a major cardiac event, patients tend to have either depression and/or anxiety related to their recovery and how to approach the changes in lifestyle being requested of them. For cardiac patients to be able to make voluntary, informed decisions about their care and recovery, they need understandable information on a variety of topics such as medication compliance, nutrition issues, correct heart-oriented exercise methods, and how to manage stress and anger.

For cardiac patients who have ongoing or residual fears concerning their recovery, psychoeducational social groups provide a safe, nurturing environment. Members get support and acceptance from their peers as well as the social group worker. Psychoeducational social groups provide an opportunity for members to give one another support and help to each other to gain an understanding from the educational materials, and integrate this information into their specific situations. As cardiac patients receive additional information on relevant topics, this reduces the threat of the unknown (i.e., surgical procedures, additional diagnostic testing, etc.). Moreover, gaining information relative to cardiac self-care helps members develop new skills, or learn new strategies to cope, that in turn enhances self-confidence.

Purpose/Goals

The main purpose of psychoeducational social groups is to expand the awareness of the medical, social, and psychological aspects of cardiac disease. A primary goal is to motivate the cardiac patient to move toward a healthy recovery process (McLennan, Anderson, and Pain 1996). Psychoeducational social groups are provided to help cardiac patients integrate and incorporate information that will help them establish a cardiac recovery plan that utilizes health and psychosocial data. Also, psychoeducational social group encourage members to make productive choices relative to the entirety of their lives.

Psychoeducational social groups also are used to challenge cardiac patients through information to accept a healthy status rather than a health status. These educational groups also increase cardiac patients' sense of commitment and determination to remain in active cardiac rehabilitation to its end, as well as effect changes in maladaptive behaviors, such as poor eating and exercise habits, poor stress management, and poor health habits such as excessive use of alcohol and tobacco use.

Some of the fundamental aspects in which psychoeducational social groups may be most helpful include: (1) helping cardiac patients in the precontemplative or contemplative stage of accepting change (in lifestyle) and their role in a change process that leads to a more healthy recovery; (2) helping patients understand other community services that will support their ongoing cardiac recovery, such as support groups; (3) helping patients, in the beginning phase of their cardiac medical and psychosocial treatment, identify barriers and obstacles to cardiac recovery, and help patients begin to develop an individualized plan of health maintenance; and (4) helping cardiac patients understand healthy uses of family support and the importance of limit or boundary setting with family, peers, and significant others in the patients' lives.

Functional Characteristics

Psychoeducational social groups generally teach cardiac patients that they need to learn information to be informed consumers and to be able to make cogent decisions about their cardiac care. Psychoeducational social groups are a necessary and important component to cardiac rehabilitation programs. Although other social group work models are helpful in motivating patients, these groups are extremely helpful in moving cardiac patients who are in a tepid, or precontemplative, or perhaps a contemplative stage of accepting self-responsibility for lifestyle changes needed to maintain a healthy cardiac recovery. That is to say, the psychoeducational social groups utilized in cardiac rehab provide the needed information that is helpful for persons needing to make lifestyle change when time is not on their side.

Furthermore, psychoeducational groups should attempt to engage members in discussions and prompt them to relate and integrate what they are learning to their specific cardiovascular problems, both psychosocially and medically. For the social group worker to avoid process issues in psychoeducational social groups is to reduce the overall effectiveness of the group context.

An example is a psychoeducational social group designed to help cardiac patients understand the need for compliance with medications. This model is designed to educate the cardiac patients about the various types of medications used in cardiac care and to help differentiate the different types (e.g., blood pressure medications, beta-blockers, calcium blockers, cholesterol medications, blood thinners); develop a basic understanding of how various cardiac and/or psychiatric medications work and interact in the human body; develop an understanding of the positive effects of specific classifications of cardiac and/or psychiatric medications; develop and hone skills in understanding the potential negative side effects for cardiac patients related to cardiac and/or psychiatric medications; enhance understanding of when and what type of conditions and negative effects should trigger the patient to seek professional help; and develop skills in being one's own advocate in asking questions of medical staff, physicians, nurses, and pharmacists when the patient does not understand or needs additional information for clarification.

Structural Characteristics

Psychoeducational social groups are generally highly structured and often follow a written protocol in the form of either a manual or curriculum. The group sessions are typically limited to set times. The social group worker takes on the role of an instructor who is leading the group discussion to help members integrate and utilize information. Although quite different in format, purpose, and structural design, psychoeducational groups need to occur in a private, quiet location to ensure confidential interaction.

Even though psychoeducational social groups can be either homogeneous or heterogeneous relative to membership sex and cardiac malady, it is suggested that cardiac psychoeducational groups should be heterogeneous in terms of membership sex but should be homogeneous in terms of cardiac issues. It is believed that this arrangement will allow for maximal interaction and allow the members to have information tailored to their specific CVD. For example, psychoeducational social groups dealing with the topic of medications would have a sexual mix in membership, but would focus content on specific cardiac disease processes such as patients dealing with post-heart-attack issues or congestive heart failure. Psychoeducational social groups have been demonstrated to be quite effective with patients dealing with comorbid disorders such as congestive heart disease and depression or anxiety (McLennan, Anderson, and Pain 1996; Lubin, Loris, and Burk 1998).

It is recommended that cardiovascular psychoeducational social groups focusing on a specific topic such as medication compliance be developed as part of a one-week curriculum of cardiac rehabilitation and lasting no longer than ninety minutes each session. The total number of group meetings should be developed relative to the aggregate of information to be shared while allowing time in each session for questions, reactions, and member responses.

Group Leadership Skills

Although cardiac psychoeducational social group workers need to have the same base characteristics and skills in terms of warmth, empathy, and genuineness, the leader needs to possess knowledge of, and skills to impart, topical information. Social group workers using this model should understand basic and complex group processes such as how individuals interact in a social group setting, how groups form and develop, and how group dynamics influence an individual member's behavior in a group context.

Also, in using the psychoeducational model, social group workers need a keen understanding of how interpersonal dynamics operate, such as how people relate to one another in a social group context and how a singular member can influence the behaviors and perceptions of others. Social group workers using a psychoeducational approach need to understand the fundamentals of teaching and how adults learn, integrate, and utilize information. Such teaching skills include organizing the content to be imparted, planning for participation in learning processes, and being able to provide information in a culturally relevant and understandable manner.

Clinical Techniques Utilized

Since individuals in the midst of a perceived crisis, such as a cardiac event or diagnosed cardiac disease in their lives, are more likely to learn through interpersonal interactions and active exploration of information rather than passive listening, the social group worker is responsible for designing active learning experiences that fully engage all participants. Four aspects of active learning can help. First, in order to stimulate active learning, the social group worker should limit the extent and duration of providing information. Thus, the leader can have more time to facilitate member discussion and integration of educational information. This is particularly germane for cardiac patients who are tepid and interpersonally shy.

In the second way to facilitate active learning, social group workers need to understand the myriad ways in which adults learn and be able to employ varying methods. People typically have definite ways they believe they learn through particular senses (i.e., visual, auditory, or experiential). Outstanding educational methods and techniques that address alternate learning style are available through the Association for Supervision and Curriculum (see Web site: http://www.ASCD.org).

Another way to actuate active learning is to encourage the patient group member to take personal responsibility for his or her cardiac recovery. That is not to say that the group members need to be blamed or shamed irrespective of dysfunctional lifestyles and practices that may have contributed to a cardiac event or disease (i.e., tobacco use, alcohol or other drug abuse, poor nutritional habits, and limited stress coping skills).

Frequently, people involved in psychoeducational social groups recall past educational experiences. Many have had negative experiences in formal or informal academic settings. Hence, the social worker needs to be sensitive to the potential anxiety that various members may experience secondary to being in an environment (i.e., the psychoeducational social group) that replicates a disturbing scene from a past educational experience. To better deal with this potential anxiety, the social group worker needs to acknowledge group members' anxiety, prevent fellow group members from scapegoating or mocking a member who is struggling to understand and utilize presented material, and demonstrate empathy to members who are showing overt signs of anxiety (e.g., withdrawal from the group, gross shyness). In essence, the social group worker needs to create an environment of learning that is prosocial, healthy, and open.

Expected Clinical Benefits and Outcomes

Generally, by using psychoeducational social groups, one can expect that the members are able to have a working knowledge of the topic presented. Also, it is anticipated that members will be able to apply and integrate information provided to their specific CVD. Using the example of a medication education group, one would expect cardiac patients to be able to articulate how their medication affects people in the general cardiovascular population as well as how the specific medication affects them. Similarly, a psychoeducational group dealing with the topic of medication adherence, would be expected to yield outcomes of increased knowledge of cardiac medication and improved understanding and identification of individual health risks related to medication adherence.

SKILL-DEVELOPMENT GROUPS

Although most skill-development social groups operate from a cognitive-behavioral format, other groups' models serve an equal purpose. Many skill-development groups also utilize some of the core concepts utilized in psychoeducational social groups. The differentiation with the skill-development social group is that a greater emphasis is placed on the development, refinement, honing, and integration of specific skill sets. Examples include the development of cardiac efficient groups and anger management groups.

Rationale for Using the Skill-Development Group Work Model

The core rationale for using a skill-development social group is to teach and allow cardiac patients to develop, master, and hone specific skills to increase cardiac output and to minimize stressors that interfere with cardiovascular recovery. Many cardiac patients enter into cardiac rehabilitation with limited to nominal skills relative to enhancing cardiac output and poor skills in self-management of anger. Given the complex nature of treating individuals having anger management difficulties, this group is covered in a separate chapter (see Chapter 11).

Purpose/Goals

The most common type of skill-development social groups for cardiac patients are coping skills training, which attempt to cultivate skills and abilities that cardiac patients need to develop for a healthier lifestyle. Although many skill-development social groups utilize psychoeducational group techniques, the primary goal of this social group is the development of skills. Skill-development social groups typically emerge from a cognitive-behavioral theoretical backdrop that assumes that cardiac patients lack needed life skills. There are a multiple number of cardiac patients who enter treatment with limited to nonexistent life skills. Therefore, the capacity of cardiac patients to develop new skills or relearn old ones is paramount for cardiac recovery.

Since many of the skills that cardiac patients need to develop, or refine, are interpersonal in nature, social groups become a natural treatment of choice. Social group members can practice skills with one another, self-assess how different individuals use the same skills, and experience positive reinforcement of the group-as-a-whole when they utilize skills effectively and efficiently.

Functional Characteristics

There is a great variation in the ways that cardiac patients meet their psychosocial, emotional, and medical needs. The particular needs being taught depend on an assessment of each specific member's characteristics, skills, and abilities. The discrete needs of the cardiac patient depend on the unique needs of the individual group member along with the specific needs being taught. In general, most cardiac patients benefit from development and enhancement of certain general skills, such as controlling negative feelings, as well as stressors and anger triggers. Skills may be highly specific to certain cardiac patients, such as anger management, cardiac exercise, and relaxation.

Structural Characteristics

Social work skill-development groups typically run for a limited number of sessions. The size of the group should be maintained at eight to ten members, with a singular group leader (if there is a co-leader, the overall number of participants should increase accordingly). The skill-development social group has to be manageable in size relative to the skills that are to be developed.

Although social work skill-development groups often incorporate aspects of psychoeducation and support, the overt goal is to build or refine cognitive and/or behavioral resources to better cope with and accommodate the cardiac patients' psychosocial environment. Psychoeducational social groups tend to focus on the development and integration of information based on which decisions can be made and action can be taken. Social support groups, to be discussed in Chapter 14, focus on providing the internal and external (environmental) supports to develop, maintain, and sustain lifestyle changes. Although a specific social group may incorporate aspects of several models, it is extremely important to maintain focus on the overall goals of the social group.

Group Leadership Skills

As with psychoeducational groups, the social group worker needs to have a thorough understanding of basic and advanced group treatment skills. These skills include an understanding of how social groups evolve and develop knowledge about the social interactions in social groups, skills in facilitating interpersonal interactions, and skills in the management of conflict. Moreover, social group workers using a skill-development model need to understand how to promote ownership of the group by the members.

Social workers using a skill-development model should be able to demonstrate the set of skills they are attempting to impart. Therefore, social group workers will need experience in appropriate modeling of the skills associated with the particular group, as well as being able to experientially help members learn discrete components of behavioral change. Additional skills needed by social group workers relate to being able to monitor the group so that no member is neglected. The social group worker needs to be aware and sensitive to how different cultural and ethnic groups accept skill-based training. Depending on the skills being developed and honed, the social worker may need additional training. For example, if the skill-development social group is related to medication compliance, the social worker will have to learn relative risks for noncompliance (e.g., medically and psychosocially).

Clinical Techniques Utilized

Specific skills and techniques used in social skill-development groups will be determined by the specific skills being taught. Although many skills are basic and require demonstration by the social group worker and monitoring and overseeing of a member's replication, such as fundamental nutrition to strengthen cardiac output, are relatively straightforward and easy for the patients once the skills are incorporated into the group member's repertoire of behaviors. Cardiac patients who have a lifetime experience of being passive, or non-assertive, may struggle greatly to stand up for themselves. Therefore, the social group worker needs to develop sensitivity to the struggles of these members, maintain a prosocial set of expectations for change in behavior, and maintain a focus and involvement with the cardiac patients that is not shaming.

There are many behavioral changes that have deeper meaning than was first thought. For example, developing assertiveness skills may have a deeper psychosocial meaning than initially expected. That is to say, in the development of assertion skills, one may elicit feelings of guilt and shame owing to a history of being victimized and not standing up for themselves. Therefore, the development of assertion skills may be incompatible with deep-rooted feelings of ineptitude, inadequacy, and/or poor self-concept. Social group workers should not immediately think that teaching new skills, or honing old ones, will lead to immediate behavioral change. Feedback from fellow group members, facilitated by the social group worker, is a healthy way to assess learning and the integration of skills as well as supporting an individual member's progress.

In using a social work skills group with cardiac patients, there are several skill development activities that are suggested for the social group worker:

- Identify and use relevant similes, metaphors, and images to communicate information to cardiac group members. Metaphors and similes are particularly effective devices for expressing information to social group members in a cogent, vivid, and tangible manner;

• Communicate persuasive messages with passion, enthusiasm, energy, and appropriate gestures to stimulate the group members to listen and act;

• Consistently promote the information in the social work skills group and maintain and notice when cardiac members follow-up or use the information provided, this allows for positive reinforcement for the members; and

• When faced with potential resistance or objections to the goals of the social skills group or the content of the specific topic being presented, anticipate and prepare persuasive strategies and techniques for overcoming barriers and obstacles.

There are some fundamental skills that the cardiac members should be encouraged to develop irrespective of the topic being addressed. Relative to enhancing these social group skills, the social group worker needs to enhance through modeling of the certain specific skills.

The social group worker needs to actively listen to the social skill group members' communication styles by observing the overt verbiage and nonverbal cues (i.e., physical reactions, gestures, and glances). The worker should practice empathic skills by really hearing what cardiac patient members are saying and attempting to understand how specific members feel. The social group worker can demonstrate attentiveness by appropriate eye contact, prosocial body posture, and verbal responsiveness. And also take time to know the cardiac group members, their interests, capabilities, and potential contribution to facilitate cooperation among cardiac patient members.

When individual cardiac members identify problem areas or situations in an attempt to integrate information being provided, the social group worker needs to probe into the core nature of the problem, assess if a similar problem has occurred in the past, and discuss how the problem was handled and the outcome achieved, that is, attempt to avoid reinventing old ways of coping.

The social group worker needs to minimize communication problems and interpersonal conflicts by modeling healthy, direct conversation. Also, by developing healthy communications within the social skills group, overall relationships are improved. When psychosocial problems occur, it is more difficult to project negative intentions on an individual with whom one has a stable relationship. The worker also needs to encourage social skill group members to depersonalize conflict by helping them objectively evaluate the feedback rather than the member. When conflict occurs in the social skills group, the social group worker needs to adopt an objective attitude and position of an equal level cardiac patient/member in search of an equitable and advantageous agreement. The social group worker needs to look for "win-win" solutions to problems and conflict areas.

The worker should allow upset cardiac patient/members to thoroughly express negative emotions (e.g., anger, disappointment, and trepidation). When negative expressions are discharged, individuals become more able and willing to work on the issue/topic. The worker needs to encourage cardiac patents to articulate their disagreement when the social group worker senses there is a difference of opinion that has not been overtly dealt with in the group context. And when one member is provoking conflict or dominating a social skill group, the social group worker needs to systematically solicit feedback from the group-as-whole by asking the members to express their thoughts on the topic.

There is a concern that social workers leading skill-development groups and teaching the same material weekly can become bored with the material and content. Therefore, to retain emotive and creative energy, as well as teaching effectiveness, social group workers can alter topics, or the leader can invite other professionals to impart various aspects of the skill development. For instance, the social group worker may bring in a pharmacist or cardiac nurse to discuss specific techniques and methods for medication compliance.

Prudence in the provision of skills requires that the social group worker has had experience in, and perhaps mastery of, the skills being taught. For example, if one is to lead a social skills development group with a topic of assertiveness training, the leader should have developed skills in this area through either training or experientially.

Expected Clinical Benefits and Outcomes

By using skill-development social groups, one can expect that the members are able to have a working knowledge of the topic and be able to demonstrate the skills attained. For this reason, often the social group worker involved in a skill development will offer a pre- and posttest to more accurately assess the inculcation of skills and techniques.

In addition, members of a cardiac skill-development social group would be expected to link practice of skills to one's reality. For example, individuals involved in cardiac skill development of appropriate exercise that strengthens cardiac output should be able to articulate how they will utilize these skills in real-time in their lives without gross defense or resistance. Moreover, cardiac patients involved in a social skills group should be able to discuss, demonstrate, and explain how the acquired skills can be used in the real world. Furthermore, the members should be able to discuss and plan how to deal with various obstacles and barriers that potentially could distract them from fully employing these skills.

Finally, one of the best ways to learn new social skills is to be able to explain and demonstrate these skills to fellow members. This method not only helps other cardiac patients, but also reinforces one's own learning and skill refinement. For example, one who has developed assertiveness skills can explain to other cardiac group members the ways and methods of using these skills in vivo. For social-skill development in assertiveness, the members should be encouraged to mentor, either formally or informally, other cardiac patients. This vicariously helps the mentor to fortify his or her own learning and practice of attained social skills.

INTERPERSONAL (SOCIAL) GROUPS

Humans are by nature social animals. Much of what occurs in the life of humans occurs within the context of social groups. How individuals manage health and sickness is socialized within the family-of-origin. The ways in which individuals act and react to one another has been inculcated within various social institutions.

Rationale for Using the Interpersonal Group Work Model

The interpersonal social group model for the psychosocial treatment of cardiovascular patients is steeped and grounded in a long history and body of knowledge of theory (Brown, Glazer, and Higgins 1983;

Leszcz, Yalom, and Norden 1985; Leiberman, Yalom, and Miles 1972). This sharply defined body of process-oriented social groups is widely diverse. As an outcome, current dynamic conceptualizations have included emphasis on the social nature and structure of human attachment, rivalry, and social hierarchies, as well as cultural and spiritual concerns (i.e., existential concerns and questions of faith). This model of social group work focuses on healing by changing basic intrapsychic (internal mental issues) and/or interpersonal (social interactions) psychosocial dynamics.

A survey of group work articles published between 1970 and 1990 suggested that many group workers who work in inpatient settings paying allegiance to some specific model of group work often claimed to use an interpersonal or interactive model (Fallon and Brabender 1992). Although the interpersonal model appears to take myriad forms depending on the patient population and the setting in which it is applied, all applications emphasize the usefulness of interpersonal learning in the group.

Although there are numerous variations of interpersonal social groups, the one promoted here is built on the clinical model developed by Yalom (1980, 1995). From Yalom's perspective, this model goes beyond symptom relief and leads the patient to gaining an understanding of the interpersonal issues precipitating it. The nonsymptomatic focus of Yalom's interpersonal social group model ensures that the contribution of the group will duplicate those of other group work modalities (Yalom 1980). The emphasis of this particular group model is relevant for individuals dealing with chronic medical problems such as cardiovascular illness, which impact the patient as well as significant others in the patients' social context.

Purpose/Goals

A central goal of the interpersonal social model in general is to foster members' development of effective and efficient social behaviors that will enable them to achieve more intimate, gratifying, interpersonal relationships. This goal is derived from Sullivanian perspective that all psychological problems, no matter how individually centered they may seem (e.g., difficulty in managing relationships while experiencing a major medical problem, such as cardiac disease), have a social undergirding. Specifically, these groups allow the cardiac patients beginning their recovery to develop healthy interactions with significant people in their lives. These groups help cardiac patients develop skills in setting healthy limits and boundaries for themselves with family, friends, co-workers, and work supervisors.

Often, cardiac patients look healthier outwardly than they really are. As such, people in general heal (recover) on the outside sooner than they do on the inside. This is true for both physical as well as emotional healing.

Interpersonal social groups use knowledge of the ways in which individuals promote change and enhance cardiac recovery. Interpersonal social groups utilize an understanding of group members' development (e.g., socialization processes) and environments (e.g., sociocultural) that have affected group members' personal views of illness and disease, and also how individuals recover, or heal, from disease processes. Developmental and environmental influences affect how individuals manage genetic and biologic vulnerability.

In addition, the interpersonal social groups focus on examination of developmental and environmental factors affecting individuals' coping and adaptive strategies relative to managing a severe disease process. As dysfunctional interactive and relationship patterns are identified, cardiac patients can work to change destructive obstacles and barriers that potentially serve to undermine cardiac recovery. By participating in an interpersonal social group, cardiac patients form mutually satisfying healthy relationships, and the skills developed in this context can be transferred to one's life outside the group.

Five major heuristics are central to all interpersonal social groups:

1. An individual's socialization, through his or her family-of-origin, school experiences, and work experiences, affects later experiences. Thus, it is understood that each cardiac group member brings his or her history to therapy.
2. Psychosocial and cognitive processes that influence behaviors, judgments, and decision making are frequently outside of the immediate awareness. As the cardiac patient begin to identify and understand various underlying socialized psychosocial dynamics that support behaviors (e.g., poor social coping) that he or she desires to change, this information can be used to develop healthier relationships and proactive social coping skills.

3. One's view of reality is based on perceptions. Individuals often make generalizations based on their view of reality that are dysfunctional and retroactive. Therefore, the interpersonal social group provides a forum to help correct various cognitive distortions that hinder habits and lifestyle changes.
4. Beyond who one's parents are, where one is born, how one is socialized in his or her family-of-origin, and disease processes that are solely genetic, everything else in one's life is a choice. Although there are many choices in life that one can make, one does not choose the possible range of outcomes. For example, a person can choose to eat unhealthy foods, but the effect of this choice is not always knowable or anticipated.
5. Individual behaviors are chosen to adapt to environments and serve to protect individuals from psychosocial harm. From this viewpoint, whether the behavior is healthy or not, behavior is the individual's best effort to cope and adapt to a particular situation. For example, behaviors such as smoking and/or excessive alcohol use or drug abuse are, in essence, the ways people have chosen to adapt and to cope.

Within the interpersonal social group model, the objects of therapeutic interest are the here-and-now (e.g., present focus) actions among cardiac group members. Of minimal significance is what happens outside the social group and what has occurred historically for the cardiac patient. There are three dynamics that social group workers need to monitor: (1) how the group-as-a-whole is functioning relative to its members and the goals of the group (i.e., group-as-a-whole dynamic); (2) the psychosocial functioning of each individual cardiac group member (intrapsychic dynamics); and (3) the ways in which cardiac group members relate to one another (i.e., interpersonal).

The social group worker conducting an interpersonal social group will tend to focus on the interpersonal dynamics and concentrate less on each cardiac group member's individual psychosocial dynamics and the workings of the group-as-a-whole.

Functional Characteristics

Although there are many applications of the interpersonal social group, a sine qua non of all such groups is the use of the here and now as a central characteristic of group treatment. The focus on the here and now is predicated on the position of Sullivan and later, Yalom (1980, 1995), that most forms of psychosocial problems have an interpersonal aspect that can be explored within the immediacy of a set of relationships found in social groups.

The interpersonal group functions as a microcosm of the way group members relate to significant people in their daily lives. As such, interpersonal social groups delve into major developmental and socialization aspects of how individuals cope with illness. In this manner, interpersonal groups allow cardiac group members to share ways of coping that have worked historically for them when confronted with major life crisis, as well as share those areas that have proven to be barriers, obstacles, and dysfunctions.

Structural Characteristics

Interpersonal social groups typically operate as open-ended (Yalom 1995). That is, new members may join the group at any point, and there are those who are terminating their involvement during any particular group session. Therefore, the life of the group is the current social group treatment session (Yalom 1980, 1995). Although specific topical content is difficult from group session to the other, the process components remain intact from one group session to the next. The size of the group should be maintained at eight to ten members, with a singular group leader.

Interpersonal social groups are relatively easy to adopt and modify because they are:

- *Reality-based and pragmatic:* This social group model is a hands-on type of group treatment. The interpersonal social group focuses on results, not abstract concepts. Its reality and result orientation is especially satisfying to a population, such as those in cardiac rehabilitation, who need immediate positive outcomes. This is particularly helpful in the beginning phase of the psychosocial aspects of cardiac rehabilitation when the opportunity for influencing and motivating patients is relatively brief.
- *Synergistic in design:* Interpersonal social groups, and physical and psychosocial cardiac rehabilitation, complement one another reciprocally, thus setting the stage for effective treatment.

Group Leadership Skills

Social group workers using this model focus on the present, noticing signs and symptoms of individuals re-creating their past in what is occurring between and among cardiac group members. The interpersonal social group worker monitors how the group members are interacting, how cardiac members are psychosocially and emotionally functioning, and how the group-as-a-whole is functioning.

The social group worker leading an interpersonal social group observes a variety of social group dynamics such as the stages of social group development, how leadership is developing and emerging in the group-as-a-whole, the relative strengths each cardiac group member brings to the group-as-a-whole, and how individual cardiac group members resistant to change interact and affect overall group functioning. Hence, the social group worker develops interventions related to his or her blend and perceptions of the group mix. In utilizing the interpersonal group model, the leader's job is to promote and probe interactions, and interventions, that assume a critical point.

Most social group workers utilizing the interpersonal social group model use the theoretical influence of the interactions proffered by Yalom (1995). Yalom recommends an adaptable approach to social group treatment, one that allows easily applied modification across the continuum of cardiac recovery. Yalom's interpersonal social model can be reconfigured in early treatment to have more predictability and structure. This model is flexible relative to the cardiac patients' outcome expectations; more structure early in treatment can be loosened (as to the group structure) as cardiac recovery is solidified.

There is always the potential that cardiac patients will revert to negative coping skills under stress at this point, and patients become more vulnerable to change.

Clinical Techniques Utilized

In their discussion on interpersonal social groups, Brabender and Fallen (1993) suggest a five-step process that guides the content of the group. First, the group worker provides members with information about the purpose (to develop and enhance interpersonal relationships that promote cardiac recovery), function (the group is a process-oriented therapy model), and structural features of the group (length of session, frequency of sessions). The social group worker explains that chronic health problems, such as cardiovascular disease, can test and strain even relatively stable interpersonal relationships. Also, the group worker explains that by working on their relationships with one another, cardiac patients can improve their relationships outside of the group. Yalom (1980) realized this orientation as extremely important, evidence that patients' knowledge of goals and working procedures of their groups enhance their overall integration and performance in the group.

The second process step of the interpersonal social group requires each member to identify some area of his or her life, which he or she can work on during that session. Yalom (1980) noted that going around the group enables the group worker to identify areas of greatest interpersonal tension so that problem areas for each member can be recognized and direction provided for further clinical exploration. Here, the group worker looks for commonality and patterns that form a member's agenda. For example, group members may highlight concerns relative to the need for interpersonal support from significant others versus an exaggerated level of support whereby the cardiac patient is not allowed to make his or her own decisions about health care. The formulation of the member agenda is seen as having immense therapeutic value (Yalom 1995).

Third, the group worker facilitates agenda fulfillment with as many members as possible. What is important at this point is for the group worker to remain alert to the possibility of utilizing and integrating as many member agendas as feasible into the context of group action. Although many member agendas are fulfilled within the interpersonal social group context, the group worker may give a member an assignment that can be used in vivo. For example, a member may have as an agenda to increase his or her assertiveness to establish healthier boundaries with a significant other (e.g., a spouse who is overly involved in the cardiac patient's medical appointments). The group worker could assign this member a limited goal to practice outside the group, such as asking the significant other to not attend an upcoming cardiology appointment.

The fourth step, the group wrap-up, consists of two retrospective analyses of the session. First, the group is analyzed by the group worker. This allows the group worker to synthesize what has occurred relative to meeting the various members' agendas as well as critique how the group-as-a-whole has responded. The social group worker's role in this discussion is to give consideration to each member's progress in the group session as well as the group-as-a-whole. At this point, the social group worker should underscore any positive comments of his or her own activity in the group session that would potentially help demystify the therapeutic process and provide a model of openness and candor. If there is a coleader, the discussion of their relationships also provides members with a demonstration of constructive interpersonal exploration.

In the second analysis, and fifth step in the process of developing and interacting in the wrap-up phase of the group session, group members are given the opportunity to bring the meeting to an end (Barbender and Fallon 1993). These final events should include an open discussion of the members' reactions to the social group worker's observations and analysis. This allows fellow group members who have not had an opportunity to speak earlier to articulate their feedback and/or synthesize understanding of the group outcomes. The group members are permitted to determine which direction to pursue because such an opportunity encourages the members to take individual responsibility. Simultaneously, the social group worker should seek opportunities to use this final phase of the interpersonal social group to support a self-review process in which cardiac group member comes to recognize more succinctly what is effective work in the group context. As an example, the social group worker may explicitly state that a given session was particularly owing to members' obvious willingness to offer one another honest, and direct, feedback relative to the management of overly involved significant others who intrude in the cardiac patient's care and decision making.

Expected Clinical Benefits and Outcomes

There are at least five expected clinical outcomes from using the interpersonal social group model with cardiac patients. First, cardiac patients will be able to identify and explain specific interpersonal areas that are problematic. Second, the group members will be able to cite areas of skill development in interpersonal relationships that need addressing. Third, cardiac patients will be able to use the group to practice (e.g., role modeling and role-playing) interpersonal skills that can be utilized with significant others outside the group context. Fourth, the cardiac group members will be able to articulate alternative ways to manage dysfunctional relationship in their lives. Finally, cardiac group members will be able to articulate ways to set healthier boundaries with family members, peers, and/or work-related supervisors.

CONCLUSIONS

CVD is a biopsychosocial problem for the patient as well as the cardiac rehabilitation staff. Cardiac patients need to address the medical aspects of their disease along with the psychosocial aspects. Cognitive-behavioral groups help the cardiac patients develop alternative ways to manage negative feelings such as depression, anxiety, and anger by challenging their own thoughts and perceptions. Through participation in psychoeducational social groups, cardiac patients can acquire information that will assist them in actively participating in their own treatment and the direction of their health care. Moreover, cardiac patients involved in skill-development groups are able to maintain a sense of independence through mastery of various skill sets. Finally, through participation in interpersonal groups, cardiac patients can enhance their communication and interactive skills with treatment professionals, peers, family members, and significant others. These interpersonal skills are particularly important when dealing with complex issues related to cardiac disease.

Chapter 5

Adherence Issues Associated with Cardiac Care: A Social Group Work Model

INTRODUCTION

One of the most difficult issues that influence both the medical and psychosocial treatment outcomes of individuals having cardiovascular disease is that of treatment adherence. Coronary artery disease is a leading cause of mortality in the United States, despite advances in understanding the underlying risk factors and drug therapy options, and the development of practice guidelines for secondary prevention. This chapter describes a motivational social group approach that enhances the potential for cardiac patients to change their lifestyle. This cardiac social group builds upon the psychoeducational and skill development core groups.

RATIONALE FOR USING THE SOCIAL GROUP WORK MODEL

Relative to cardiac medical compliance, Miller and Rollnick (1991) were among the first to study factors that increase patient commitment to cardiac care. They found that many patients fail to meet their clinical treatment goals because of poor physician adherence to guidelines, poor patient compliance, and comorbidities that require modifications to management plans. Their analysis found that by increasing the intensity of medical involvement improved cardiac patients' compliance and commitment to positive cardiac outcomes.

Social Group Work with Cardiac Patients
© 2007 by The Haworth Press, Inc. All rights reserved.
doi:10.1300/5739_05

Beyond medical factors that influence compliance, the presence of discernible psychosocial or mental health issues also affects cardiac treatment and outcomes. One of the chief factors is the co-occurrence of depression with cardiac disease. Research over the past two decades has shown that *depression and heart disease* are common companions and worse, each can lead to the other. It appears now that depression is an important risk factor for heart disease along with high blood cholesterol and high blood pressure. In an analysis conducted by the National Institute of Mental Health (NIMH), it was found that of 1,551 people who were free of heart disease, those who were depressed were four times more likely to have a heart attack in the next fourteen years than those who were not (NIMH 2002).

In many cases, depression and heart disease go hand in hand. When this happens, the presence of the additional illness is frequently unrecognized, leading to serious and unnecessary consequences for patients and families. Although depressed feelings can be a common reaction to heart disease, clinical depression is not the expected reaction. For this reason, when present, specific treatment should be considered for clinical depression even in the presence of heart disease. Appropriate diagnosis and treatment of depression may bring substantial benefits to the patient through improved medical status, enhanced quality of life, a reduction in the degree of pain and disability, and improved treatment compliance and cooperation.

Most obviously, if an individual does not comply, symptoms may not be relieved or the disorder may not be cured. However, not complying may have other serious or costly consequences. Noncompliance is estimated to result in 125,000 deaths due to cardiovascular disease (such as heart attack and stroke) each year (AHA 1998).

PURPOSE/GOALS

The overriding purpose of conducting a motivational enhancement social group is to improve the cardiac patient's commitment to making potentially lifesaving changes. Since individuals vary in their level of understanding concerning their cardiovascular disease, patients will vary as to how seriously they take their role in cardiac recovery. Some individuals are so well defended that either they minimize the seriousness of their cardiac illness or they are in denial about both the disease and their responsibility and involvement in cardiac recovery. Hence, there is a delicate psychosocial balance between improving the patient's understanding and commitment to change strategies versus inducing additional fear that would have a "chilling effect" on the patient's willingness to accept the reality of the cardiac disease and promoting the patient's involvement.

Not only does nonadherence add to the cost of medical care, it can also worsen the quality of life. For example, missed doses of certain medicines can lead to optic nerve damage and blindness in people with glaucoma, to an erratic heart rhythm and cardiac arrest in people with heart disease, and to stroke in people with high blood pressure. Not taking all prescribed doses of an antibiotic can cause an infection to flare up again and may contribute to the emergence of drug-resistant bacteria.

FUNCTIONAL CHARACTERISTICS

The social group that deals with enhancement of motivation in cardiac patients functions as both an informational and process group. The social group worker needs to provide needed information concerning the seriousness of having cardiovascular disease while affording the cardiac patient the opportunity to internalize this information and utilize it to enhance his or her willingness to change (i.e., commit to a cardiac recovery plan of action). To this end, the social group worker utilizes both cognitive-behavioral techniques as well as Socratic questioning that helps the cardiac patient internalize the information and commit to change.

To ascertain the level of commitment and motivation, cardiac patients and their families need to be assessed relative to where they are in terms of motivation and stages of change (e.g., willingness to make changes). Ideally, the initial assessment prior to involving the cardiac patient needs to be accomplished in an assessment/individual evaluation of the cardiac client, along with his or her family, prior to involving the participants in a motivational enhancement social group process. In practicality, the evaluation of the cardiac group member occurs within the context of a social group process.

After the initial cardiovascular event, cardiac patients need to be assessed to rule out medication nonadherence. This process should occur within a social group context to gain the input of fellow members and the social group worker. Cardiac group members will be assessed relative to motivation (i.e., willingness to change) as well as their commitment to change. Upon evaluation, the cardiac patient will be intervened based on his or her willingness to change (e.g., accept an appropriate level of change to move to a higher, and more, healthy level of change).

STRUCTURAL CHARACTERISTICS

As soon as the cardiac patient is medically cleared to participate in a social work group, the patient needs to be involved in a motivational enhance (ME) social group (Miller and Rollnick 1991). These groups are neither overtly professionally directed nor are they assertive. Cardiac patients' should be interviewed and assessed individually prior to entry in this group in order discern the patient's level of understanding of his or her cardiovascular condition, as well as to discern the level of change to which the patient is committed. Furthermore, this initial interview allows the social group work to gain an understanding of the concerns and fears that confront and confound cardiac rehabilitation. This process also gives the social group worker an opportunity to assess the level of family social support for cardiac change.

Although ME social groups with cardiac patients can be either homogeneous or heterogeneous relative to membership gender and cardiac disease, it is suggested that these groups should be heterogeneous in terms of membership gender, age, and cardiac issues. It is believed that this arrangement will allow for maximal interaction and allow the members to have information tailored to their specific cardiovascular disease.

The ME social cardiac group should be open-ended to allow the individual cardiac patient whatever time and exposure individually needed to improve his or her motivation. However, the social group worker needs to monitor each cardiac patient on an ongoing basis to help identify and assess how the patient motivation has shifted. As the cardiac patient moves toward increasing self-responsibility for his or her cardiac recovery, commitment to ongoing cardiac care and adherence, the social group worker will move toward terminating the patient from the group. The ME cardiac social group should meet at least weekly for one to two hours. Given the intensity of technically helping to motivate individuals, the group needs to maintain a core of not more than twelve patients during any given session (Miller and Rollnick 1991; Rollnick, Mason, and Butler 1999).

GROUP LEADERSHIP SKILLS

Among the basic social group skills utilized to help members form, process, and utilize what is gained in group with in vivo situations of the cardiac patient's life, the worker needs to have specific skills in underreacting to cardiac patients who are resistant to change because of mental health issues such as depression, anxiety, and anger. The social group worker needs to have a replete understanding of how defense mechanisms work (i.e., to keep individuals psychosocially and emotionally safe), understanding the difference between internal versus external defenses (e.g., suppression of emotions versus projecting of emotions), and the social group worker needs to have a sophisticated understanding of clinical resistance and alternative ways to help frame resistance in positive terms. The following are general clinical guidelines of how to use resistance in healthy ways that promote motivation and commitment to change and ongoing compliance with both medical and psychosocial recommendations.

Some of the suggested social group worker skills in using the ME model include but are not limited to the following:

- Understand the cardiac patient's frame of reference.
- Filter the cardiac patient's thoughts so that statements encouraging change are amplified and statements that reflects status quo are minimized.
- Elicit for the cardiac patient statements that promote prosocial and positive change such as expressions of problem recognition, concerns, desires, health goals, intentions to change, and the ability to change.
- Match the processes used in theory to the stages of change, and ensure that they do not move beyond the state where the cardiac patient is medically, emotionally, and psychosocially.

- Use ongoing expressions of acceptance and affirmations that the cardiac patient can change and improve his or her life situation.
- Promote the concept of "free will" to empower the cardiac patient to involve himself or herself in key medical decisions.
- Affirm the cardiac patient's "freedom of choice" and his or her right to self-direction as well as self-determination.

CLINICAL TECHNIQUES UTILIZED

The social group worker needs to have clinically specific skills in using the following techniques: Socratic questioning, motivational interviewing, an understanding and working knowledge of the stages of change, fear management techniques, and use of the group-as-a-whole to enhance goal-setting as well as decreasing resistance and defense.

Socratic Questioning

Socratic questioning is a qualitative way of going through a process of self-discovery. All questions are designed to solicit from the cardiac patient what his or her goals and desires are relative to their cardiac disease. Although directive in its method, the social group worker serves this group as a consultant seeking information from the cardiac patient. The process allows the cardiac patient to be genuinely heard, not simply listened to, or patronized.

Table 5.1 provides the social group worker with a template relative to specific interventions based on the cardiac patient's stage of change (e.g., degree of acceptance of having a cardiac disease as a reality). Irrespective of the stage of change, group members can be mixed within the same group. The social group interventions would differ based on the individual cardiac patient's stage of change. That is to say, the interventive methodology directed to the individual cardiac patient is unique, irrespective of the change stage the members are in, that all can benefit.

Motivational Interviewing

Motivational interviewing (MI) is a patient-centered counseling developed by Miller and Rollnick (1991) to facilitate change in health-

TABLE 5.1. Readiness to Change Assessment and Matching

Stage of Change	Service Task	Treatment Processes	Intervention
Precontem-plation	Grappling with reality of cardiac disease	Consciousness-raising; beginning of understanding	Basic; use of Socratic methods and reflective listening
Contem-plation	Grappling with reality of cardiac disease	As above, plus emotional arousal, self-evaluation	Basic; use of Socratic methods; cognitive-behavioral cost-benefit analysis
Preparation	Mix of grappling with reality of cardiac disease, plus acceptance	Emotional arousal, self-evaluation, commitment to treatment adherence	Increase use of cost-benefit analysis and cognitive-behavioral techniques
Action	Acceptance of cardiac disease as a reality	Commitment, reward, countering; environment control; full linkage with helping professionals	Reinforcement; support; encouragement
Recycling	Reversion to questioning cardiac disease as a reality	Based on assessed stages of change to which the patient has regressed or recycled	Use of clinical reminders and positive reinforcement of what the patient has presented as clinical material for acceptance of the cardiac disease

related behaviors (e.g., accepting and entering into cardiac recovery). MI uses a directive method to approach the enhanced intrinsic motivation for behavior change by working with and resolving ambivalence (Miller and Rollnick 1991; Rollnick, Mason, and Butler 1999). Originally developed to work with problem drinkers (Miller and Rollnick 1991), MI has now been used and tested with a broad range of health behavior including cardiac diseases (Rollnick and Butler 2003). Research has qualitatively shown that the use of confrontation actually solidifies the patient's resolve to not make health changes.

There are seven core techniques inherent in MI that are helpful in group treatment of cardiac patients:

1. Encouraging the cardiac patient to share his or her goals about cardiac outcomes (e.g., that the cardiac patient wants to live a healthy life)

2. Eliciting from the cardiac patient the fears and concerns relative to his or her cardiac condition and possible outcomes (e.g., that the cardiac patient fears an impending death)
3. Encouraging the patient to express empathy by using reflective listening to convey understanding of the cardiac patient's perspective and his or her underlying psychosocial drives
4. Helping the patient identify any discrepancies between the cardiac patient's most deeply held values and the patient's current behavior (i.e., solicit ways in which current unhealthy behaviors, such as refusing to eat "heart smart" food or involvement in cardiac exercise protocol, conflict with the patient's stated goal, such as living longer)
5. Holding the cardiac patient responsible for his or her self-management and involvement in medical decision making
6. Circumventing resistance by only responding with empathy and understanding rather than confrontation
7. Supporting self-efficacy (i.e., self-mastery) by building the cardiac patient's confidence that change is not only a possibility, but also a positive probability

Patient Assessment of Stages of Change As an Ongoing Tool

Most individuals, at one time or another in their lives, reach a point when they know that something in their lives has to change, and that the cardiac patient and respective family members have to be the ones to change it. Be it spiritually, mentally, emotionally, or physically, the status quo is no longer satisfying their needs, and it is time to do something about it. When it comes to one's self-image, it is often a grueling and difficult task to make a change; however, because the thoughts that have "fed" behaviors for so long are deeply ingrained in one's psyche, the habits of thought are hard to break.

Psychologists Prochaska, Norcross, and DiClemente (1994), among others, have developed a theory about the process of change, and the process by which one can be effective at implementing change in his or her life. This model is called the transtheoretical model, and it involves a number of steps by which people have been professionally and successfully treated and taught to manage their problem behaviors through behavior modification. An ongoing assessment of

where the cardiac patient is in the process of making positive com-
mitments and changes, this model considers the next level of change
process, as well as assesses potential obstacles and barriers in the cardiac patient's way of reaching the next level, and ultimately success.

It is noteworthy that not all individuals involved in the change process are at the same stage at any given point in time. In some cases,
the cardiac patient may revert back to an earlier level of psychosocial
change before he or she can in fact move on. In this way, the process
of change propounded by Prochaska and DiClenente (1994) is best
conceptualized as a circular rather than linear. When the cardiac patient reverts back to earlier, and perhaps more regressive, stages of
change and commitment, the social group worker needs to maintain a
prosocial direction, helping the cardiac patient move to the next specific stage as soon as it is acceptable for the patient.

Although motivational interviewing started from a basis of clinical
empiricism, several theoretical models, most notably the transtheoretical model of change, which is described later, and dissonance
theory proffered by Festinger (1957) have been borrowed to provide
an academic framework.

The basic principle that underpins most models of change in health
behavior is that individuals hold a range of representations about their
problematic symptoms and behaviors. At one extreme are individuals
who are stoic or in denial, and neglect themselves and their disease
symptoms. Conversely, there are those who display abnormal illnesses
or disease behaviors and in reality adopt a sick role (i.e., "cardiac
cripple" versus "cardiac patient in recovery"). Models of behavioral
change include the notion that there are at least two major components to an individual's readiness to change. These are importance/
conviction and confidence/self-efficacy (Rollinick and Butler 2003)
encapsulated in the adage "ready, willing, and able." *Importance* refers
to why change is needed. The concept includes the personal values and
expectations that will accrue from change. *Confidence* refers to the individual's belief that they have the ability to master behavior change.
The theorems of change place these concepts into more practical, usable terms that social group workers can use in practice.

Hence, MI works on both of these dimensions by helping the cardiac patient articulate his or her rationale as to why it is important for
him or her to change, and by increasing self-efficacy, which promotes

enhanced self-confidence and thereby minimizes potential compromises in treatment and ultimate noncompliance.

Often there is confusion between and fusion of MI and the transtheoretical model of change developed by Prochaska and his colleagues (Prochaska and DiClemente 1992; Prochaska, Norcross, and DiClemente 1994). The transtheoretical model of change breaks down the concept of readiness to change into six stages, from not even thinking about change to maintaining change once it is made. One implication of this model is that for each stage, helping behaviors are particularly constructive.

MI and the transtheoretical model of change are developed separately but do coalesce. MI had no theoretical base and the transtheoretical model filled only some of the vacuum. MI is the type of process that is useful for individuals who are in the early stages of determining whether a change is needed. The following stages of changes developed by Prochaska and DiClemente (1992) are not necessarily linear, but tend to occur in a process similar to identifying where the cardiac patient is relative to his or her commitment to change. Levels of commitment and change are influenced by psychosocial shifts within the patient, external (intrapsychologic) as well as impacted upon from the cardiac patient's psychosocial context in which he or she lives. These stages of change are the following:

1. *Precontemplation:* At this point, the cardiac patient is not even ready to think or ponder over a change in his or her lifestyle.
2. *Contemplation:* Here, the cardiac patient is beginning to think about making a change, but there is great ambivalence to be dealt with.
3. *Commitment:* The cardiac patient is ready to think about making a planned change; unwittingly, this is done through an internal "cost-benefit" self-assessment.
4. *Preparation/action:* The cardiac patient has developed a plan for change and is ready to actuate the change in healthy ways.
5. *Action:* At this change stage, the individual is committed. The cardiac patient is physically, emotionally, and spiritually ready to embark on a journey by which the individual will improve his or her life, and they follow a plan of action. This leads to implementing change.

6. *Maintenance:* At this stage, the individual holds his or her head higher. He or she has more self-confidence. The danger at this stage, after the individual has made some big changes, is that one may slide into unhealthy coping methods. At this stage of change, the goal is about ensuring that the change is behavioral and becomes habitual.

Promoting change, especially change that presumably affects an individual's perception of his or her lifestyle, can be emotionally and physically daunting. The concept of "change" has unwittingly acquired a negative connotation in our society. The historical ways in which medicine has played a paternalistic role has made change even more complex. Through the use of MI techniques and the stages of change as an ongoing assessment tool, many individuals experiencing cardiovascular disease are serving, and are feeling empowered, by playing the role of "informed consumer." The decision-making burden is shifting to the well-informed cardiac patient. But this shift is not without hesitancy on the part of the consumer and his or her family. This is due in part to the fact that the consumer, along with well-meaning family members and significant others, have to increasingly accept responsibility for decisions and judgments made.

Fear Management

There are several factors that potentially serve as either a barrier or an obstacle to the cardiac patient's move through the stages of change. Here, the social group worker is dealing with helping the cardiac patient manage his or her natural fears relative to dealing with cardiac diseases. Fears and concerns that are well meaning, but not accurate, need to be dealt with directly. Fears that emanate from hearsay, or even "urban legend," need to be confronted directly to not sustain delusional thinking or false beliefs. Helping the cardiac patient to manage fear ensures that medical and psychosocial changes will occur and improve decision making and judgments as well as improve cardiac outcomes. Derived from Dennis O'Grady's (1998) seminal work, these fears include, but are not limited to, the following:

Fear of the Unknown

Even with a mentally competent cardiac patient, typically, his or her life experiences do not prepare them for making decisions that may affect the course, literally and figuratively, of their life. Understanding cardiovascular disease continues to be quite technical and not necessarily user-friendly for the patient and family. Some research has shown when individuals perceive themselves to be in good health, they want increasing involvement and control of their health care. But, when the situation of an individual's health is complicated, individuals want to follow more closely the advice of the expert. As a result, fear of the unknown can paralyze an individual.

Fear of Failure

Typical questions that confront cardiac patients are related to human decision-making errors irrespective of the health information being provided by the experts. Unfortunately, individuals expect to get everything right the first time, instead of taking their time to work things out and getting them right at some time.

Fear of Commitment

Fear of making a decision is why some individuals do not set firm goals or accomplish what they set out to do. They are afraid to focus on what they want versus what they need in terms of cardiac health care. They use the excuse that they will be trapped in a particular decision, when there are often other options available as additional information is provided. Cardiac patients should be honest with themselves and commit to a few simple and heartfelt goals, before moving to larger decisions that have more risk attached to them.

Fear of Disapproval

Some might call this the fear of rejection. This is particularly true for individuals who are in need of dependent approval from others, and have difficulty in going against what significant others or families may want for them. If an individual makes a change, somebody will likely disapprove. It is not uncommon for several people in the cardiac patient's social network to feel this way.

Fear of Success

Contrary to the "fear of disapproval" is the fear of making the correct, well-thought decision about an individual's cardiac care. Some individuals will exercise their informed decision making and self-determination, and the end result will be a positive outcome. When people get through the changes and are feeling good, they sometimes feel guilty for feeling good. Individuals often trace this guilt back to being taught that they are selfish and egotistical for taking care of themselves.

The Stage of Medical Crisis: A Potential Fear

When a cardiac patient is presented with having to make a decision or judgment under some major time constraints, this heightens a sense of crisis and stress for them. This sense of crisis—usually very emotional—is a wake-up call, telling an individual that he or she is confronting a need for change.

The Stage of Hard Work: Another Potential Fear

This is the stage that most cardiac patients tend to tolerate and embrace. This is, in essence, the stage that allows the patient to fully exercise his or her self-determination relative to decision making and judgments that ultimate affect cardiac outcome. Often this involves hard mental work. An individual may take classes, read books, and network with business contacts. There is a sense of control in this stage—one is working hard trying to figure out the solution to the crisis.

USE OF THE GROUP-AS-A-WHOLE

The group-as-a-whole can serve as an invaluable source of feedback and negative critique that can improve the cardiac patient's decision making, commitment to change, and ultimate compliance. The group worker using this model facilitates the use of the group-as-a-whole to help individual cardiac patients self-assess where they are in making and committing to change that is durable and lasting. Often, cardiac patient group members may not heed the advice and feedback of professionals, but will listen to and hear the feedback of individuals in a similar situation. This is particularly true when the stakes are psychosocially high, and potentially affect an individual's mortality.

The social group worker in this type of treatment needs to use both reflective listening and reflective feedback of the group-as-a-whole (i.e., what the social group worker gleans as the group's feedback to a specific cardiac patient). This allows the individual group member sufficient time to arrive at a decision, judgment, or conclusion that fits him or her best, relative to the potential outcomes of psychosocial and medical cardiac outcomes. Here, the social group workers need to be mindful about not unduly promoting their own thoughts at the expense of the cardiac patient.

The general nature of the group-as-a-whole allows for consensus building while providing needed help and encouragement for actuating a particular decision and judgment concerning cardiac care and treatment options. In addition, the group-as-a-whole serves as a "sounding board" that the individual cardiac patient can utilize to maintain a reality base upon which cogent decisions and judgments can be made. Finally, the use of the group-as-a-whole can offer the needed support that can energize cardiac patients in positive directions.

EXPECTED CLINICAL BENEFITS AND OUTCOMES

An individual in this social group can experience several expected outcomes. These outcomes serve to refine the cardiac patient's decision making concerning both psychosocial and medical outcomes. These benefits include the following:

1. Increase in prosocial, proactive decision making concerning cardiac treatments
2. Enhancement of the cardiac patient's ability to make cogent judgments about cardiac treatments
3. Improvement in overall adherence to follow-up with cardiac care in a systematic manner
4. Development of healthy support systems that provide cardiac patients an emotional platform upon which decisions and judgments about an individual's cardiac care can be made

5. An ongoing reality check for cardiac patients regarding the decisions and judgments that need to be made relative to cardiac psychosocial and medical treatment
6. An improvement in the cardiac patient's overall commitment to be informed about psychosocial and medical decisions

CONCLUSIONS

Nonadherence is always a potential barrier to successful treatment. Adherence becomes increasingly more challenging when the patient has a comorbid disorder such as depression and cardiovascular disease. Through the group process, utilizing clinical methods that help the patient self-assess his or her own readiness to change compliance can be enhanced. By participating in a group process that promotes positive change, ongoing individual self-assessment as to one's readiness to change (e.g., confronting one's own fears) and responsible decision making, the patient may increasingly make healthier choices. In this manner, the social group provides knowledge and information integration that will enhance cardiac patients' overall adherence and ultimate cardiac recovery.

Chapter 6

Social Work Group
for Heart Attack Patients

INTRODUCTION

A heart attack is an event that can result in permanent heart damage or death. It is also known as a *myocardial infarction,* because part of the heart muscle (*myocardium*) may literally die (infarct). A heart attack occurs when one of the coronary arteries becomes severely or totally blocked, usually by a blood clot. When the heart muscle does not receive the oxygen-rich blood it needs, it will begin to die.

The severity of a heart attack usually depends on how much of the heart muscle is injured or dies during the heart attack (CDC 2005a). A heart attack is an event that results in permanent damage or death to part of the heart muscle. One's chance of surviving a heart attack depends on the medical treatment that is given within the first hour of the heart attack. Immediate treatment for a heart attack should always include professional emergency medical intervention, including a call to 911, if the patient lives in an area with such access. While waiting for help to arrive or on the way to the hospital, patients are often told to begin chewing *aspirin*, a blood clot inhibitor. It is thought that taking aspirin while experiencing a heart attack can decrease the risk of death by about 25 percent (CDC 2005a,b).

The American Heart Association (AHA) estimates that in 2004, more than one million Americans will suffer a heart attack (AHA 2005b). About 700,000 of these will be first-time heart attack sufferers, while about 500,000 will be people who had previously had a heart attack.

Social Group Work with Cardiac Patients
© 2007 by The Haworth Press, Inc. All rights reserved.
doi:10.1300/5739_06

Before a heart attack, the person may experience an episode of *cardiac ischemia,* which is a condition in which the heart is not getting enough oxygen-rich blood. This is often accompanied by *angina* (a type of chest pain, pressure, or discomfort), although *silent ischemia* shows no signs at all. Severe, multiple, or lengthy episodes of cardiac ischemia or unstable angina can be a warning of imminent heart attack.

Depending upon the severity of both the attack and of the subsequent scarring, and how rapidly the person gained access to medical service, a heart attack can lead to:

- Full recovery, occurring in the majority of patients
- Heart failure, a chronic condition in which at least one chamber of the heart is not pumping well enough to meet the body's demands
- Electrical instability of the heart, which can cause a potentially dangerous abnormal heart rhythm (arrhythmia)
- Cardiac arrest, in which the heart stops beating altogether, resulting in *sudden cardiac death* in the absence of immediate medical attention
- Cardiogenic shock, a condition in which the damaged heart muscle cannot pump normally and enters a shocklike state that is often fatal
- Death

A heart attack is not the same thing as cardiac arrest, even though many people use the terms interchangeably. Cardiac arrest occurs when the heart actually stops beating and pumping blood, usually due to a malfunction in the heart's electrical system (*ventricular fibrillation*). The term *massive heart attack* is also mistakenly used to describe cardiac arrest, but they are not the same thing. A heart attack may lead to cardiac arrest, but these are separate events.

Although a heart attack may be the result of a number of chronic heart conditions, the trigger for a heart attack is often a blood clot that has blocked the flow of blood through a coronary artery. In most cases, the cause of the blood clot is linked to *atherosclerosis,* also known as "hardening of the arteries."

Heart attacks may also be caused by a *coronary artery spasm,* a temporary constriction of an artery in the heart.

RISK FACTORS AND CAUSES OF HEART ATTACKS

The AHA estimates that in the United States in 2005, approximately 700,000 people will have a heart attack for the first time (AHA 2005a,b). Age, genetics, and lifestyle factors (e.g., diet, activity levels, and smoking) play a role in heart attack risk. Scientists are continually researching these and other potential risk factors. Centers for Disease Control and Prevention researchers (CDC 2005a,c) report that people with cardiovascular disease whose arteries are clogged with fatty plaque—which tends to rupture—may be at higher risk of heart attack than patients with *calcification,* a process that makes plaque harder and more brittle, forming a crust over plaque formations. The risk of plaque rupture appears to increase in the morning hours, which may explain why more heart attacks occur between 6:00 a.m. and noon.

People with chronic kidney disease tend to have high blood pressure, which places added stress on waste-removing filters in the kidney (nephrons). Uncontrolled high blood pressure also contributes to heart disease through a process known as *remodeling,* where there is enlargement and weakening of the heart's left ventricle (left ventricular hypertrophy) and increased risk of heart attack. Research has found that heart attack survival decreases even with mild to moderate kidney disease.

People with high levels of a certain type of lipoprotein called Lp(a) in the blood may be at an increased risk of heart attack. Research has found that high Lp(a) levels may increase a person's risk of heart attack over a ten-year period by as much as 70 percent. In addition, people with *metabolic syndrome* have been found to have twice the risk for heart attack and stroke, when compared to people without the syndrome. The characteristics of metabolic syndrome are elevated fasting blood glucose levels, abdominal obesity, high LDL ("bad") cholesterol levels, high triglyceride levels, and high blood pressure.

Patients whose parents have had a heart attack before the age of sixty years have a higher risk for developing CVD at a young age. Studies have found that patients (average age of nineteen years) whose parents had early heart attacks can have thicker artery walls and worse artery function than is normal for their age. Researchers suggest that a genetic cause may be responsible, stressing the need for healthy life-style changes for patients with a family history of early heart attack.

Genetic research has also shown that people with one particular estrogen gene are three times more likely to have a heart attack than are people without the variant. All people—both men and women—have the gene, but only a small number have the variant that increases heart attack risk.

The role of race in heart disease is currently being explored. In the year 2000, the Jackson (Mississippi) Heart Study was launched to better understand why black Americans have a higher mortality from heart disease than white Americans do. Sponsored by the National Institutes of Health, it is modeled after the famed Framingham Heart Study (2004). More than 6,000 black American men and women (ages 35 years to 84 years) in Jackson, Mississippi, are being studied. A combination of physical examinations and questionnaires are being used to document and establish risk factors for CVD in black Americans.

RATIONALE FOR USING
THE SOCIAL GROUP WORK MODEL

A heart attack is not a one-time, one-moment occurrence. It is a process that builds up over a period of few hours. With each minute that goes by, less oxygen reaches the surrounding heart muscle, and the risk of permanent damage rises. Therefore, someone's chance of surviving a heart attack depends on the treatment that is given within the first hour of the heart attack. The vast majority (about 90 percent) of heart attack patients who reach the hospital alive survive the event (CDC 2005a).

In addition, a heart attack is an unnerving event that triggers fear, ambivalence, and, often, a direct correlation to one's own mortality. Especially with males, the presenting heart attack maybe a follow-up of a "silent heart attack" (i.e., one in which the patient did not recognize as a heart attack and may have rationalized as indigestion or other gastrological events).

PURPOSE/GOALS

The general purpose of a social group designed to address heart attack recovery is to normalize the event and encourage cardiac patients to deal with the reality of the cardiovascular event. Also, the cardiac patient needs to understand the progressive nature of the disease and develop individualized ways to address the heart attack in a healthy, prosocial manner.

It is possible to reduce one's risk of developing atherosclerosis (hardened arteries) in one or more coronary arteries, thus eliminating a major risk factor in heart attacks. In fact, it is easier to prevent future damage than it is to heal damage that has already been done. The AHA (1988) recommends that people have their blood pressure, body mass index (BMI), waist circumference, and pulse checked at least once every two years, beginning at the age of twenty years. Cholesterol tests and glucose tests are to be made at least once every five years. Such risk factors, according to the AHA, can be used to estimate the risk of developing heart disease within a ten-year period.

Although people cannot change their age or family medical history, there are risk factors that people can change. Because it has been proven that the buildup of plaque is increased by certain behaviors, recommended changes include:

1. *Improving one's cholesterol ratio:* A person's total cholesterol level (which includes LDL cholesterol, HDL cholesterol, and triglycerides) should be no more than 200 mg per deciliter and no more than five times the HDL level. Key strategies for reducing levels of total cholesterol, LDL cholesterol, and triglycerides are to eat a heart-healthy diet and to exercise regularly. If these strategies do not reduce total cholesterol levels, a physician may prescribe cholesterol-reducing drugs (e.g., statins). Strategies for increasing levels of HDL cholesterol include eating monounsaturated fats in moderation, decreasing the amount of saturated fat, limiting alcohol use, and starting an exercise program.

2. *Regular exercise:* Exercise can be an excellent tool in both the prevention of heart disease and for improving quality of life for heart patients. Physically, it can slow or even reverse the process of atherosclerosis, as well as lower blood pressure and reduce cholesterol levels. Emotionally, it can reduce levels of stress and depression.

3. *Achieving and maintaining a healthy weight:* Obesity and being overweight are major risk factors for a host of serious health conditions, including CVD, high blood pressure, diabetes, heart attack, and stroke. Some weight control methods include limiting calories, increasing activity, counseling, medication, and surgical interventions.

4. *Having a heart-healthy diet:* Modern research has consistently supported the idea that health is largely determined by what people choose to eat. Certain B-vitamins and minerals have been shown to be helpful to heart health. Omega-3 fatty acids found in certain fish (e.g., tuna, salmon, and sardines) may keep arteries healthy and elastic. Saturated fats and tropical oils (palm and coconut oil), however, have been shown to be harmful, because they can speed up the development of CVD, atherosclerosis, and obesity.

5. *Quitting smoking and staying away from all secondhand smoke:* Tobacco smoking is a major cause of CVD and cardiac arrest. According to the United States Centers for Disease Control and Prevention (CDC 2005a), from 1995 to 1999, nearly 450,000 people in the United States died prematurely from smoking. Of these, nearly 150,000 deaths were attributed to cardiovascular diseases and nearly 125,000 were attributed to lung cancer. The CDC (2005a) also estimates that secondhand smoke was responsible for more than 35,000 deaths from ischemic heart disease (and 3,000 deaths from lung cancer) annually during the same five-year period.

6. *Controlling blood pressure:* Individuals with high blood pressure (hypertension) are at a greater risk of heart attack and other problems resulting from cardiovascular disease. Current research suggests that hypertension can bring on changes in genes involved in heart function. This contributes to a process known as remodeling, in which there is enlargement and weakening of the heart's left ventricle (left ventricular hypertrophy). Cells involved in heart muscle contraction become impaired and eventually self-destructive, leading to heart failure. Hypertension can be controlled through taking blood pressure medications, self-monitoring, eating a heart-healthy, low-salt diet, and engaging in regular exercise. People are also encouraged to have regular checkups with their physician.

7. *Controlling diabetes:* People with diabetes may be more likely to develop heart-related diseases. However, recent studies have shown that people with diabetes may reduce their risk of heart attack by taking

acarbose, a medication that helps control blood sugar levels by slowing carbohydrate digestion. The medication has been shown to be effective with nominal negative side effects.

FUNCTIONAL CHARACTERISTICS

This social group functions as both a process model and educative model. The social group worker is in a position to provide cogent information about the causes of heart attacks as well as alternative ways to prevent further medical complications. In addition, the social group worker utilizes process skills to help cardiac patients incorporate information on heart attacks and helps the patients to apply this information to his or her personal situations.

This social group should provide a forum to help clients understand what a heart is and how it is manifested differently in males versus females. Also, the members should be able to develop an understanding of how heredity, family biologic history, lifestyle, nutrition, and psychosocial dynamics affect the chances for heart attack, as well as the ways in which one can minimize these factors. Cardiac patients who have had a heart attack are then positioned to seek important information from cardiac care staff and cardiologists that will allow them to make informed decisions relative to their care.

In addition, this type of social work group is process-oriented relative to how heart attacks are experienced by the patient and his or her family. As it is with other CVDs, the quality of a patient's life should be discussed in relation to how having a heart attack can be managed medically, emotionally, and psychosocially. This type of social group has a focus on demystifying the disease and normalizing the experience so that cardiac patients will not feel alone in their struggle, and can deal with the reality of the disease, its treatment, and how it affects one's life and lifestyle. That is, cardiac patients should be allowed to share their experiences of dealing with a heart attack, how it has affected them as individuals, how the heart attack has affected their family, and how they have developed alternative ways to cope that are not shaming or limiting.

STRUCTURAL CHARACTERISTICS

It is suggested that this social group be conducted on at least a weekly basis with not more than eight to ten cardiac patients. Irrespective of age, the mixture of clients is both male and female. The following areas need to be addressed to aid in helping patients make lifestyle changes:

- *Learning and practicing stress management techniques:* Stress, excessive anger, and fatigue can lead to high-risk practices such as overeating, smoking, high blood pressure (hypertension), and a lack of exercise. In addition, chronic stress may be a direct contributor to poor heart health because it increases blood pressure that could become permanent. Anxiety has also been linked to an increased risk for future health problems in men who have suffered a heart attack.
- *Recognizing and treating chronic depression:* Depression has been linked with a higher risk of developing high blood pressure, heart disease, and having a heart attack. Depression is associated with heart disease in several ways, including a risk of abnormal heart rhythms (arrhythmias), alteration of the amount of blood flowing to the coronary arteries, increased risk of blood clots ("sticky" platelets), and increased risk of sudden cardiac death. A recent study of the antidepressant drug *sertraline* found that it was a safe and effective therapy in patients having a recent heart attack or unstable angina. It has also been shown to have anticlotting properties.

It is unfortunate that up to two-thirds of postattack patients do not make lifestyle changes. It is estimated that up to one-third of fatal heart attacks could be prevented with the proper preattack medical treatments and lifestyle modifications (CDC 2005a). Even after one heart attack, the chances of avoiding future attacks can be increased with appropriate preventive care. People who have had a heart attack, or are at risk of having one, are encouraged to remember that their lifestyle choices can have a major impact on their heart health. Patients should always consult their physicians before making any changes to their diet or activity levels.

Much attention has been given to the possible benefits of moderate alcohol consumption in lowering the risk of heart attacks and heart disease in general. At this point, medical experts do not recommend that nondrinkers begin drinking alcohol for better cardiovascular health. Research is still being done to clarify the relationship between alcohol and the heart. However, findings in recent years have suggested that moderate alcohol consumption may offer some people a degree of protection against heart disease. Moderate drinking is defined as not more than one drink per day for women and not more than two drinks per day for men. One drink is equal to the following: 12 ounces of beer or wine cooler, five ounces of wine, or 1.5 ounces of 80-proof liquor. Whether or not to drink is something patients should discuss with their physicians. More important, however, is to follow established, proven wellness strategies. The earlier in life a patient modifies his or her habits, the better the chances of lowering or even eliminating certain risk factors for heart attack.

GROUP LEADERSHIP SKILLS

As with other social groups for cardiac patients, the social group leader needs to develop a comfort level in dealing with and discussing potentially life-threatening issues such as a heart attack, as well as being familiar with the various causes of heart attacks. The social group worker also should promote a social context of sharing of feelings and risking the expression of fears, whether rational or not. In addition, the social group worker needs to be able to help, encourage, and facilitate individual members in the following ways:

- Promote empathy (i.e., attempting to place oneself in another situation), not sympathy (e.g., feelings of sorrow), among cardiac patients who have suffered through a heart attack.
- Help the patient develop an understanding of the medical conditions that lend themselves to the potentiality of having a heart attack.
- Help the cardiac patient accept the heart attack as a reality for the individual member (irregardless of heredity, lifestyle, and health habits).

- Facilitate the cardiac patient in developing an understanding of male versus female psychosocially experienced heart attacks, as well as how family members experience the event.
- Create a therapeutic clinical environment for the expression of feelings about having experienced a heart attack.
- Promote the discussion of thoughts (e.g., worry about developing another heart attack; guilt about how the member may have not attended to his or her body's signals of cardiac problems) and feelings (e.g., fear of having a follow-up heart attack; concerns and fears about one's own mortality and the fragile nature of human life).
- Develop an understanding of how the human heart works, what a heart attack is, and how individuals who have had heart attacks typically, psychosocially experience the condition.

Therefore, the social group worker needs a thorough understanding of how the human heart functions, medical and psychosocial variables affecting heart attack recovery, and how males versus females deal with potentially life-threatening diseases (i.e., heart attack). In addition, the social group worker needs to be able to empathize with individuals who have experienced a life-threatening condition, and what is considered the norm for males versus females after experiencing a heart attack.

CLINICAL TECHNIQUES UTILIZED

Beyond fundamental social group work skills, the social worker needs to help groups develop a sense of cohesion. The social worker leading a social group dealing with heart attacks will need to develop skills and abilities in the following areas of clinical practice: (1) a thorough understanding of what heart attacks are and how heart attacks physiologically and psychosocially manifest themselves; (2) an understanding of how individuals respond to potential life-threatening illnesses (e.g., fear, anxiety, depression, and/or anger); (3) an understanding of and empathy for the effects of a heart attack on individual group members; (4) an understanding of how males versus females develop, cope with, and manage heart attacks; (5) alternative ways for cardiac patients diagnosed with a heart attack to utilize external resources; (6) an understanding of how typical families deal with potentially life-threatening illness such as heart attacks; and (7) if the social group worker is unable to respond to requested information, the social group worker needs to develop an appreciation and understanding of when and how to refer cardiac patients diagnosed with heart attack to another professional who can address their concerns in a timely manner.

EXPECTED CLINICAL BENEFITS
AND OUTCOMES

The most important outcomes for cardiac patients who have experienced a heart attack within the context of the social group are that individual patients develop the following:

1. An increased awareness of how to detect cardiac symptoms that signal a potential heart attack
2. A basic understanding of how heart attacks manifest themselves in males and females
3. A basic understanding of the typical course of a heart attack
4. Increase in feelings of self-mastery and gain hope through obtaining relevant information
5. Individual understanding of the patient member's unique heart attack process
6. Understanding the overall effects that a patient having a heart attack has on the family
7. Through an understanding of human heart attacks, their function, and progress, the cardiac patient will be able to make informed life and medical decisions and
8. Through a more comprehensive understanding of heart attacks and their typical progression, the cardiac patient could be less dependent upon others, which would lessen the likelihood of becoming a "cardiac cripple" (a victim).

CONCLUSIONS

Heart attacks have a devastating psychosocial and medical effect on the patient. Often, an individual who has suffered through a heart attack feels isolated and alone. Moreover, there is a tendency for the individual to become withdrawn and retreat from their supports. By involving the cardiac patient in a social group context, the heart attack experience can be normalized and fears explored. The social group serves to provide cogent information about heart attacks, obtain factual information about the typical course of management of heart attacks and allow individual members to process their unique experience.

Chapter 7

Social Group Work
for Heart Failure Patients

INTRODUCTION

Heart failure is a serious condition in which the heart's pumping action is compromised. In the early stages, heart failure may not have any symptoms. In the later stages, the patient may have severe symptoms because their weakened heart is unable to pump enough oxygen-rich blood with each contraction to satisfy the body. These symptoms may include shortness of breath (*dyspnea*) that initially occurs only during exercise, and later even while at rest. Heart failure is a chronic and complex condition. By itself, heart failure is not considered a disease. Rather, it is the result of other conditions that damaged the heart. These other conditions include diseases of the coronary arteries that lay on the surface of the heart, heart valve disorders, high blood pressure, and damage to the heart muscle itself.

According to the American Heart Association (1998), heart failure affects about 5 million Americans, with more than half a million new cases diagnosed every year. Interestingly, while the incidence of other cardiac diseases remains stable or varies only slightly, the incidence of heart failure has increased significantly over the past three decades (CDC 2005a). This is because of the aging population and physicians' increased ability to treat other cardiac diseases. In the 1970s, high blood pressure was the leading cause of heart failure. Today, *coronary artery disease* is the leading cause because of the increased survival due to treatments such as bypass surgery and balloon angioplasty.

Social Group Work with Cardiac Patients
© 2007 by The Haworth Press, Inc. All rights reserved.
doi:10.1300/5739_07

In spite of its name, heart failure does not mean the heart has completely stopped, which is the case when someone has gone into *cardiac arrest*. Heart failure means the heart is not operating efficiently and therefore must work harder to make up for the shortcoming. For example, the heart may pump more frequently to compensate for its weakened pumping ability, or the size of its chambers may increase, especially the left ventricle.

The longer the heart must overwork to compensate for its shortcomings, the more its pumping ability is damaged and the more likely that serious pumping failure will result. Before a pumping failure occurs, however, various physical changes may take place in the heart and throughout the body as a result of the heart failure.

Heart failure may be defined by how it affects patients. The New York Heart Association (2002) has developed a system that defines heart failure by the functional limitation it imposes on the patient. These levels are as follows (with approximate percentage of patients):

- *Class I:* No obvious symptoms, no limitations on patient's physical activity (35 percent of heart failure patients)
- *Class II:* Some symptoms during or after normal activity, mild physical activity limitations (35 percent of heart failure patients)
- *Class III:* Symptoms with mild exertion, moderate to significant physical activity limitations (25 percent of heart failure patients)
- *Class IV:* Significant symptoms at rest, severe to total physical activity limitation (5 percent of heart failure patients)

The American College of Cardiology and the American Heart Association (2005) have developed a way to define heart failure that groups patients by their risk of developing heart failure. This system is useful because it helps physicians design a therapeutic approach to heart failure. The AHA/ACC stages are:

1. *Stage A:* The patient is at high risk for heart failure, but has no heart abnormalities.
2. *Stage B:* The patient has structural abnormalities of the heart, particularly the left ventricle, but no symptoms.
3. *Stage C:* The patient has past or present symptoms associated with heart failure.
4. *Stage D:* The patient has end-stage heart disease, requiring specialized treatment (e.g., continuous intravenous [IV] drug ther-

apy, left ventricular assist device, heart transplant) or severely symptomatic heart failure.

RATIONALE FOR USING
THE SOCIAL GROUP WORK MODEL

Beyond being diagnosed with a heart attack, heart failure has an extremely ominous sound to those diagnosed with this type of cardiac disease. As stated, heart failure itself is not considered a disease. Rather, heart failure is the product of another condition that damaged the heart muscle. Thus, the development of heart failure is intimately connected to the prevalence of other cardiac diseases. From a psychosocial frame of reference, the diagnosis of heart failure needs to be explained to the cardiac patient in a way that allows him or her to place it in context. Although life-threatening, most forms of heart failure can be treated and maintained, so as to not worsen the condition.

Comparing the incidence and course of heart failure between Caucasian and black Americans is provocative. Studies have found that in Caucasian patients, heart failure most often occurs as a result of CVD, such that CVD develops directly into systolic heart failure. Black Americans, however, tend to progress more gradually from hypertension (high blood pressure), to heart wall thickening, to diastolic heart failure, and finally to systolic heart failure. Statistics also show black American heart failure patients to be younger and more likely female, as compared to Caucasian patients. In addition, black Americans with heart failure are more likely to be diagnosed with hypertension and diabetes. Although some studies have shown that black Americans have higher heart failure mortality rates than whites, other studies have shown similar survival rates between the two racial groups. The reasons for these differences are still being investigated.

Research has uncovered a significant difference in the way heart failure appears in older patients, according to a study sponsored by the National Heart, Lung, and Blood Institute (NHLBT 1999). The study examined the rates and types of heart failure found in more than 5,800 individuals aged 65 years and over. Incidences of heart failure were greater among men in the trial than among women and increased progressively with age. In addition, heart failure rates were higher among patients with a history of diabetes, atrial fibrillation (a heart rhythm disorder), or mild kidney failure (NHLBT 1999, 2002).

PURPOSE/GOALS

The overall purpose of this group is fourfold. First, it is to help the cardiac patient deal with the reality of having heart failure. Second, it is to help the cardiac patient understand what heart failure is in general terms, and specifically how heart failure affects the individual and his or her family and significant others, both medically and psychosocially. Third, it is to help the cardiac patient destigmatize the illness for himself or herself relative to a specific CVD. Finally, it is to help promote and enhance one's knowledge of heart failure, in order to promote informed consent and voluntary decision making among patients relative to the course of their treatment.

FUNCTIONAL CHARACTERISTICS

The cardiac heart failure group functions both as a didactic and process model that allows cardiac patients and their respective family members to gain a fundamental understanding of what heart failure is and how it affects patients and their respective family members. Also, this social group provides alternative ways on how heart failure is developed, as well as how heart failure is influenced by heredity, lifestyle, nutrition, and psychosocial dynamics. Cardiac patients are then positioned to seek important information from cardiac care staff and cardiologists, which will allow them to make informed decisions relative to their care.

This type of social work group is also an interactive process in its orientation relative to how the heart failure diagnosis is experienced by the patient and his or her family. The quality of a patient's life is discussed in relation to how heart failure can be managed both medically and emotionally. Finally, this social group has a focus on destigmatizing and demystifying the disease so that the cardiac patient can deal with the reality of the disease, its treatment, and how it affects one's life and lifestyle.

STRUCTURAL CHARACTERISTICS

Since heart failure is usually a chronic condition that has taken years to develop and worsen, treatment for heart failure is generally designed for four purposes: to improve any symptoms, to slow progression of the heart failure, to prolong survival, and to increase prosocial coping skills in treatment decision making. In addition, physicians may choose to treat the underlying conditions that contributed to the heart failure while social group workers may choose to empower the cardiac patient with alternative methods to manage the effects both psychosocially and emotionally.

It is suggested that the heart failure social group be conducted weekly and be open-ended so that cardiac patients can enter the group at any point and receive the didactic information and avail themselves to the interactive process elements.

The following topical format is recommended to maximize group treatment elements. Most patients diagnosed with heart failure are advised to make lifestyle changes, regardless of the severity of their condition. The following seven topical areas represent the core of what the typical cardiac patients having heart failure should address:

Lifestyle Changes

These may include modifying their diet, limiting salt intake, achieving and maintaining a healthy weight, learning and practicing stress management skills, quitting smoking, and getting regular exercise, depending on the severity of the illness.

Limiting Physical Activity Until Approved by One's Physician, and Then Stay As Active As Possible

Heart failure patients who exercise regularly typically show significant improvement, whereas heart failure patients who are inactive show a clear decline. In studies, tai chi (an ancient Chinese workout involving slow, relaxing movements) has been shown to benefit patients living with heart failure. However, exercise in any form is beneficial. Patients should consult their physician before beginning an exercise program.

Scheduling Relaxation and Rest Periods
Throughout the Day

An assessment of how cardiac patients manage free time and re-laxation is necessary. Given the nature of a technologically sped-up life in today's' culture, the world is not necessarily divided into thirds (i.e., eight hours of sleep, eight hours of work, and eight hours of dealing with one's own interest and attending to family expectations).

Avoiding Excessive Fluid Intake

Since excessive fluid intake can have a negative effect on the man-agement of one's heart failure, alternative ways to maintain an appro-priate fluid intake in general, and specific to the cardiac patient group member, should be discussed. Avoiding excessive salt intake, which may contribute to fluid retention, should be highlighted and discussed relative to the cardiac patient's lifestyle.

Diary/Journal Keeping

Keeping a diary of one's daily weight, and notifying one's physi-cian if there is a weight gain of three or more pounds in a single week (which may indicate fluid retention and the need for an immediate change in treatment). Patients experiencing weight loss in spite of what appears to be adequate calorie intake should also discuss their situation with their physician. A study has found that some patients with heart failure may need to adjust their diet to meet increased en-ergy needs.

Limit Alcohol Intake

Patients with heart failure should be reminded to always consult their physician before taking any over-the-counter medicines, vita-mins, or herbal supplements. Alcohol and illicit substance should be strongly discouraged.

Medication Compliance

Depending on the nature of the underlying damage or malfunction that led to heart failure, medications may be prescribed to reduce the heart's workload, effect remodeling, counter abnormal hormonal levels, increase blood flow, widen vessels, or eliminate excess water from the body. Because the medications have different effects, they may be used in combination under the guidance and oversight of the patient's cardiologist.

GROUP LEADERSHIP SKILLS

Beyond a fundamental understanding of group process as to how groups develop and evolve, the social group workers who lead a heart failure group will need the additional skill sets such as being well-educated and versed on the etiology of heart failure, how it progresses, and what the general outcomes are for cardiac patients with this condition; understanding the psychosocial aspects of heart failure relative to how this condition manifests itself and progresses; a keen understanding of how this condition affects significant others and families; an understanding of how lifestyle affects heart failure and the patients medically and psychosocially; being able to manage stigma as related to the client's condition, as well as being able to articulate alternative methods to deal with stigma; understanding their limitation relative to dealing with myths and misconceptions about the condition of heart failure; and understanding how to make a referral to other cardiac health providers for additional evaluation of the patient who is unable to manage the group process.

In sum, the social group worker needs to develop an intellectual and emotional group comfort level in dealing with a serious, possibly fatal, condition such as heart failure. The social group worker needs to be able to empathize with the cardiac patient while maintaining a focus on prosocial, healthy ways to psychosocially manage this condition.

Finally, the social group worker needs skills in helping cardiac patients maintain a realistic understanding of the condition of heart failure, and also must be comfortable in allowing cardiac group members to process their own understanding of the condition. The social group worker needs to be open to allowing cardiac patients to explore the meaning of this condition, and finally, should be able to afford the cardiac patient a therapeutic context in which to explore emotions, thoughts, and outcome expectations.

CLINICAL TECHNIQUES UTILIZED

Beyond the basic social group work skills, one needs to help group members develop a sense of cohesion. The social group worker leading a heart failure group will need to develop skills and abilities such as an ability to provide information that is pragmatic and relevant to the cardiac patient diagnosed with heart failure; gain a thorough understanding of what heart failure is, how it generally progress, and psychosocial ways that cardiac patients can minimize the negative effects; impart an understanding of how individuals respond to potentially life-threatening illnesses; promote an understanding of and empathy for the stigma associated with this condition; explore alternative ways for cardiac patients diagnosed with heart failure to utilize external resources; provide an understanding of how typical families deal with a potentially life-threatening illness; and extend an appreciation of when and how to refer cardiac patients diagnosed with heart failure to professionals who can address their concerns in a timely manner.

The social group worker needs to develop skills in facilitating group interaction aimed at providing members with a safe, healthy environment to share concerns, feelings, fears, and thoughts about having heart failure.

EXPECTED CLINICAL BENEFITS
AND OUTCOMES

The most important outcomes for cardiac patients involved in a cardiac heart failure social group are that individual patients develop the following:

1. Basic understanding of how the heart failure manifests itself
2. Basic understanding of the progressive nature of heart failure
3. Increase in feelings of self-mastery and gain of hope through obtaining relevant information
4. Individual understanding of his or her specific heart failure, and its typical course
5. Understanding the overall effects of how having a heart failure affects the family

6. Through an understanding of the human heart failure, its function, and progress, the ability to make informed life and medical decisions
7. Through a more comprehensive understanding of heart failure and its progression, the capability of being less dependent upon others, which lessens the likelihood of becoming a "cardiac cripple"
8. Willingness to share anxieties, fears, and concerns about having heart failure

CONCLUSIONS

Being diagnosed with heart failure is not a death sentence. In most cases, the cardiac patient diagnosed with heart failure can improve his or her cardiac output and thus prolong their life. Negative emotional reactions can hamper cardiac recovery and prolong the disease process. With social groups, the cardiac patient can develop healthier coping skills and make a transition to a healthier lifestyle.

Chapter 8

Social Group Work with Patients with Implanted Cardiac Devices

INTRODUCTION

Since the early 1950s, cardiac researchers have been developing and refining implantable devices that help regulate the human heartbeat and/or stimulate hearts that medically are functioning at a lower level than is healthy. Although in early times, many of the devices either did not work or did not work well (Bax et al. 2005a).

A pacemaker (or *artificial* pacemaker, so as not to be confused with the heart's natural pacemaker) is a medical device designed to regulate the beating of the heart. The purpose of an artificial pacemaker is to stimulate the heart when either the heart's native pacemaker is not fast enough or if there are blocks in the heart's electrical conduction system that prevent the propagation of electrical impulses from the native pacemaker to the lower chambers of the heart, known as the ventricles. The first human implantation was made in 1958 by a Swedish team using a pacemaker designed by Rune Elmqvist and Åke Senning.

A biventricular pacemaker, also known as CRT (cardiac resynchronization therapy), is a type of pacemaker that can pace both ventricles (right and left) of the heart. By pacing both sides of the heart, the pacemaker can resynchronize a heart that does not beat in synchrony, which is common in heart failure patients. CRT devices are shown to reduce mortality and improve quality of life in groups of heart failure patients.

The heart failure pacemaker is implanted under the skin of the chest and connected to three leads (soft insulated wires) that are inserted

Social Group Work with Cardiac Patients
© 2007 by The Haworth Press, Inc. All rights reserved.
doi:10.1300/5739_08

through the veins into the heart. The device is battery-powered and delivers tiny electrical pulses to both ventricles, which makes them beat in a synchronized way. These tiny impulses are small and usually not felt.

CRT, in combination with a complete program of therapy, has proven to improve the quality of life for many patients by reducing symptoms of heart failure, increasing exercise capacity, and allowing them to resume many daily activities. It is not a replacement for drug therapy. It is recommended that anyone choosing to receive CRT also continue taking medications as determined by a physician.

Typically, the patient's cardiologist may use certain criteria to determine whether an individual is a potential candidate for CRT (Bax et al. 2005a), such as (1) the patient has ventricular dysynchrony, that is, the two lower chambers of the heart are not beating together and are unable to pump blood to the body effectively; (2) the patient's medications do not adequately treat the symptoms, and the patient continues to have a poor quality of life; (3) the patient's heart failure has been classified by the doctor as Class III or IV (New York Heart Association 2002); (4) the patient's heart is not able to pump blood effectively (also called low ejection fraction); or (5) the patient still has symptoms even though he or she has been taking the maximum amount of medication the doctor has prescribed.

For some patients, CRT has been shown in clinical trials to improve the ability to exercise and perform other physical activities, improve quality of life, and improve the New York Heart Association (2002) functional class (Classes III, IV—the heart failure classification system, developed by the New York Heart Association widely used in the diagnosis of heart failure).

Now, there is growing clinical evidence to support the wider use of implantable cardioverter-defibrillators (ICD) as a primary intervention for certain patients with serious ventricular arrhythmias. These devices were initially developed in the 1970s, with the first human use in 1980. Original devices had a singular therapeutic option of defibrillation only; the generator was implanted when the thoracotomy was required. With advances in technology, the units have become more compact and can be implanted pectorally. Moreover, antitachycardia pacing, low energy synchronized cardiac high-energy defibrillation shocks, can be given via a singular lead.

Nowadays, ICD implantation is technically straightforward and is only more complicated than pacemaker implantations. Attention to asepsis is necessary, and prophylactic antibiotics are generally used. In part, ICD implants are generally conducted with sedation. Most cardiac patients can be discharged to home within twenty-four to forty-eight hours after implantation following posttransplantation of the device. Cardiac patients are typically followed-up to four to six weeks postimplant, then at three to six months intervals (Bax et al. 2005b).

RATIONALE FOR USING
THE SOCIAL GROUP WORK MODEL

Sudden cardiac death is a common problem, and increasing numbers of cardiac patients are surviving a first episode of a ventricular arrhythmia. Patients who survive either ventricular fibrillation or sustained ventricular tachycardia have further episodes, which in some cases are fatal. Until recently, arrhythmic drugs have been the standard of treatment for patients having ventricular arrhythmia, but despite using the best appropriate medical treatment, arrhythmia recurrence rates last years in most cases.

Individuals typically have fear and trepidation concerning any invasive or quasi-invasive operative procedure, especially when there is a foreign object implanted into one's body. This fear factor is seen as quite normal.

The general rationale for using a social group work model is that it is conducive to dealing with a number of cardiac patients who have been determined to benefit from some sort of implantable device (ID). In general, patients are interested in gaining an understanding of the individual effects and experience of those who have been involved in ID. Typically, individual cardiac patients who have been referred for ID have myriad trepidations about having an implantable cardiac device in their body relative to purpose, effect, and experience. There is a certain level of fear and discomfort about having such a medical device implanted. From an experiential perspective, cardiac patients truly want to know how the device is to be helpful, and what the potential drawbacks are, along with the experiences of other patients who have had such a device implanted.

PURPOSE/GOALS

Therefore, the overarching purpose of having a social group devoted to ID is to normalize and destigmatize the process, as well as to afford potential cardiac patients the opportunity to seek in vivo experiences and information from those who have had such procedures.

The major goal when conducting a social group work, which deals with implantation devices (e.g., deliberator, pacemaker, CRTs, ICDs) is to achieve the following:

- Increase the cardiac patient's understanding of the rationale for having an ID device relative to individual's specific cardiac disease
- Decrease and help the cardiac patient explore his or her fears, trepidations, and concerns relative to accepting an implanted device
- Help the cardiac patient accept the need for an ID relative to his or her cardiac needs
- Help the cardiac patient explore his or her feelings about such procedures as well as the impact this will have on the specific patient and on the family in general
- Gain an understanding of the limits and risks as well as the positive benefits for having the ID
- Empower the cardiac patient to make an informed decision relative to this medical procedure

FUNCTIONAL CHARACTERISTICS

The main functions of this social group are threefold. First, the group should be designed to provide adequate and concise information about IDs and the medical need for such procedures. Second, the group needs to be focused on the development of information so that the cardiac patient can make an informed decision. Finally, the group needs to be emotionally supportive to the cardiac patient.

Hence, the social group dealing with IDs has to simultaneously be able to deal with specific content issues concerning the procedures as well as providing an emotionally corrective experience for the cardiac patient and the group-as-a-whole.

Given the nature of this group, the social group worker needs to feel comfortable to seek additional information for the members as needed and have a willingness to invite other professionals into the group context who can address specific topical areas.

STRUCTURAL CHARACTERISTICS

Given the nature of the social group focused on members needing to hear from "those who have gone before them" in terms of having an implanted device, it is wise for the social group worker to have an open-ended group. This allows members who have had a cardiac device implanted to be able to express their thoughts, feelings, and understanding of the experience. Also, having a mix of cardiac patients, both who have already had a cardiac device implanted along with those medically suggested and referred for an ID, allows the patients to express real concerns and experiences. Only those cardiac patients who have had an ID procedure and those anticipating an ID should be the singular inclusion criteria. This type of social group is conducive to a mix of cardiac patients who are either male or female. For the best results, in terms of facilitating group interaction and cohesion, the size of the group needs to be limited to eight to ten patients.

Although the social group focused on cardiac device implantation needs to be structured, it works best if it is ongoing, so new members can enter or leave at any point in the group process. In this way, new members can benefit from peers who have already undergone the ID procedure.

GROUP LEADERSHIP SKILLS

Social group workers leading a group devoted to cardiac device implantation should have a good working knowledge of the various cardiac diseases and conditions that makes one a candidate for this procedure. The social group worker needs to have a functional understanding of the cardiac disease that warrants an ID procedure. Moreover, the social group worker needs to gain an understanding of how IDs work. The social group worker needs to understand, and be able to articulate, the benefits and risks of having an ID procedure.

Beyond the working of social group work procedures, the social group worker also has to be in a clinical position to dispel myths and legend. Often, cardiac patients have only fundamental knowledge about how the heart works, and less understanding of how cardiac diseases affect cardiac functioning. In some cases, cardiac patients anticipating an ID procedure are misled by those for whom the procedure did not work, or did not work well. Thus, the social group worker is in the unique position of having to minimize worry by helping the patient focus on the most likely outcome of a successful cardiac device implantation.

CLINICAL TECHNIQUES UTILIZED

The social group worker will need to employ educational, experiential, didactic, and process methods. It is recommended that the information provided to cardiac patients who have been referred for an implantable cardiac device be provided along with showing the devices to be implanted. Being able to touch and hold specific devices makes the experience real. The information needs to focus on the need for such devices along with helping the cardiac patient understand both the benefits and risk of these devices. In addition, the cardiac patient needs to be given information about the devices along with the potential complications. The social group worker needs to be able to deal with questions and provide information that is at once technical, but also readily translated into terminology that the typical cardiac patient can understand.

Furthermore, the social group worker needs to monitor the process aspects of the group-as-a-whole as well as specific members. In doing so, the social group worker will be able to deal with the cardiac patients' full range of emotion (i.e., fear and uncertainty of the unknown). He or she needs to be able to elicit question in an environment that is warm, friendly, and open to all levels of questions.

Cardiac patients who are referred for an implantable cardiac device need to be offered written material that explains the operation of the device and highlights how to discern if the device is not working, potential complications of the device, and when to seek immediate medical attention. Cardiac patients should be able to take the written information with them when they leave the group context and be encouraged to raise questions and concerns in subsequent group sessions.

EXPECTED CLINICAL BENEFITS
AND OUTCOMES

There are myriad curative aspects in having cardiac patients interact in a social group that allows members support, understanding, and nurturance. The most important clinical outcomes are as follows:

- Increase in the heart patient's understanding of how implantable cardiac devices work relative to the human heart and its ultimate function
- Improvement in understanding how the implantation procedures work and how they are monitored
- Decrease in the cardiac patient's fears and trepidations about cardiac implantable devices
- Develop a sense of being informed and being able to provide a consent based on the most current technological data available:
  —This implies the cardiac patient will make a cost-benefit self-assessment of the pros and cons of having this procedure as well as assessing the pros and cons of not having the suggested procedure
  —This also fosters a sense of free-will and self-determination in decision making
- Gaining the necessary support from significant others and key family members in honoring the decision made by the cardiac patient

CONCLUSIONS

Cardiac patients who have been evaluated as needing an implantable device are typically unnerved about having a mechanical device in their body. There is accompanying fear and trepidation. The social group work process can help educate the cardiac patient as well as provide needed support. Similarly, the social group affords the cardiac patient a forum to help normalize the process and assuage fears through the group-as-a-whole.

Chapter 9

Social Group Work
with Heart Transplant Patients

INTRODUCTION

Heart transplantation is the most sophisticated and complex surgical procedure conducted at this time. Often, an individual's heart failure condition progresses to the point where transplantation is medically considered as the final step in helping the cardiac patient live and maintain a healthy lifestyle. Typically, as cardiac patients diagnosed with heart failure medically decompensate, transplantation is assessed as the only viable option (Psychosocial Aspects of Transplantation 2002). This option is most often experienced by the cardiac patient as a fear-induced choice.

Patients referred for consideration of cardiac transplantation begin a complex process that involves a number of distinct phases and many challenges. Patients begin with the diagnosis of end-stage heart disease.

Adults who require cardiac transplantation usually have a primary diagnosis of end-stage cardiovascular disease (44 percent) or cardiomyopathy (46 percent). A small number are referred for transplantation due to congenital heart disease, valvular heart disease, or failure of a previous graft. Congenital heart disease is the most common indication for transplantation in young children, and cardiomyopathy is the most common diagnosis in older children (CDC 2005a).

Social Group Work with Cardiac Patients
© 2007 by The Haworth Press, Inc. All rights reserved.
doi:10.1300/5739_09

The number of centers performing heart transplants and the number of procedures performed increased exponentially during the 1980s and leveled off in the early 1990s. As summarized by Crone and Wise (1999), The Registry of the International Society for Heart and Lung Transplantation (ISHLT) has reported data pertaining to heart transplantation for over twenty years. The registry is combined with data from the United Network for Organ Sharing (UNOS), and includes the majority of centers located outside the United States. The number of heart transplant procedures performed per calendar year peaked in 1994, with 4,466 heart transplants reported that year from about 300 centers. This number has slightly declined over the past few years, with 3,646 heart transplants reported for 1998 (Hathaway et al. 1999). UNOS reports that 2,182 of these procedures were performed in the United States in 1999, where 142 centers compete for a limited number of donor hearts. Despite the limited number of procedures performed, the number of candidates registered for heart transplantation increases daily. UNOS currently reports this number at over 4,000 (UNOS 2005).

Cardiac transplant teams are increasingly challenged to support the growing number of candidates who wait for a suitable donor. The median waiting time is now over 200 days, but the candidate's blood type, weight, and status play a role. In 1998, candidates with blood type O had the longest median waiting time (299 days), and blood type AB had the shortest (68 days). Although males constitute 75 percent of cardiac transplant candidates, they usually wait longer than females (229 days versus 150 days) because of the necessity of donor-recipient weight matching (Olbrisch and Levenson 1991; UNOS 2005). Notably, death rates on the heart transplant waiting list have decreased over time. However, despite an overall decrease in death rates, patients listed as status I had much higher death rates than those listed as status II (671 [67.1%] versus 163.2 [16.3%]). The death rate per 1,000 patients was 461.5 in 1989 and dropped to 192.2 in 1998 (Levenson and Olbrisch 1993).

One-year survival following heart transplantation in adults is 85.2 percent and five-year survival is 67.9 percent (Levenson and Olbrisch 1993). Graft survival and patient survival are almost exactly the same, as it is seldom possible to replace a failing graft. Long-term survival rates are highest for recipients 35-49 years of age. There is little difference in survival between status I and status II candidates as general groups. Patients at highest risk include those requiring a ventilator or left ventricular assist device (LVAD) prior to transplantation, those with previous transplants, a diagnosis other than CVD or cardiomyopathy, and those of older age. Donor risk factors in heart transplantation include longer ischemic time, donor age (optimal age is 11-34 years), and female gender (Hathaway et al. 1999). Black recipients had lower survival in comparison to other minority groups and white recipients. Patient survival at five years was 71 percent for white patients and 58 percent for black patients (Levenson and Olbrisch 1993). In the pediatric population, the patients at highest risk are the youngest. Other risk factors include older donor age and the need for mechanical support prior to transplantation (Hathaway et al. 1999).

The causes of death following heart transplantation differ according to the time period. In the immediate postoperative period, problems such as allograft dysfunction and bleeding may lead to death. Within the first year, infection and acute rejection are common and expected problems and may become life threatening. After four years, coronary artery vasculopathy and nonlymphoid malignancy are the most common causes of death (Hathaway et al. 1999). There is a constant fall-off in survival over time, with a constant mortality rate of approximately 4 percent per year.

RATIONALE FOR USING
THE SOCIAL GROUP WORK MODEL

The treatment of last resort for certain very serious life-threatening cases of heart failure is heart transplant. Replacing the human heart in appropriately identified cardiac patients has proven quite effective. A heart transplant typically is a lifesaving medical treatment for advanced heart failure. However, donor hearts are scarce and limited, since the donor is diseased, and other concerns, including organ rejection, limit the use of this option. Typically, candidates for heart transplants are younger than sixty-five years and have healthy vital and functional organs other than the heart; donors have no other life-threatening conditions or diseases.

Current research indicates that emotional and physical cardiac rehabilitation is helpful for cardiac patients by increasing their endurance, energy level, and capacity to perform activities of daily living. A number of changes occur in the cardiovascular system posttransplantation. These changes include modifications to the typical cardiac rehabilitation program. For example, the response of an individual to exercise is different in terms of heart rate.

There are similar issues involved with pretransplant patients and posttransplant patients. For cardiac patients referred for transplantation, there is fear and concern prior to and after heart transplantation. Prior to transplantation, cardiac patients are fearful about the potentialities of death, organ rejection, and medical complications. After heart transplant, there are fears about dying, medical complications, and organ rejection as well as the myriad mixed feelings including anxiety and worry.

Therefore, the use of a social group model that includes both pre- and posttransplant patients is recommended. Those preparing for transplantation can learn from those transplanted, and those who have undergone transplantation can address concerns that crosscut issues involving all cardiac patients.

PURPOSE/GOALS

Beginning with their initial contact with and evaluation by the transplant team, patients and families move through a relatively standard series of events and phases of the transplant process. These include evaluation for candidacy as a potential transplant recipient, the wait for a suitable donor organ, the surgery, and postoperative recovery period, and long-term adjustment to posttransplantation.

The events and phases can vary considerably in their duration, depending on factors such as the severity of the patient's illness, the local and regional availability of organ donors, and the requirement that candidates accrue specific amounts of time on the transplant waiting list before being transplanted. However, the general sequence of the events and time periods is similar among all types of solid organ transplant candidates and recipients.

A number of typical health experiences arise or continue to be important from a psychosocial perspective during each phase of the heart transplant process. This lends clinical credibility for mixing those who have been transplanted with those awaiting transplant. Some of these experiences are unique to specific phases (e.g., continued deterioration of function of the native organ during the waiting period, or physical rehabilitation in the early posttransplant phase). Others are present across most or all phases (e.g., quality-of-life [QOL] issues), although the central elements of concern to patients and their families in these areas vary over time.

The psychosocial issues that arise in organ transplantation span the entire transplant process, from evaluation for transplant candidacy through the long-term posttransplantation period. There are a variety of assessment and intervention options available, but transplant teams need to tailor those options to the resources available, and also to the unique needs of their specific patient populations. Attention needs to be paid to new strategies for patient care using telecommunications. The benefits of attention to psychosocial issues justify the costs; to the extent that patients' needs are recognized and addressed across the transplant experience, long-term physical health outcomes—*the ultimate goal of transplantation*—are more likely to be realized.

The overarching purpose of a social group with pre- and posttransplant patients is to educate, support, and process heart transplantation. The pretransplant patients need to gain an understanding of what to expect; the posttransplant patients need to understand their psychosocial and medical limitations. Both pre- and posttransplant patients need support and empathy. They need to clinically process their feelings and concerns about cardiac transplantation. Typically, there are myriad and mixed feelings and concerns prior to and after transplant.

The context of a social group provides a stable and safe clinical environment for both pre- and posttransplant patients to identify feelings and stressors, and challenge underlying negative thoughts and perceptions. By affiliating with one another, transplanted heart patients and those awaiting transplant can develop relationships and social connections that allow each other to develop trust among themselves concerning the medical and psychosocial transplantation process.

Education of the patient and family is also extremely important. Patients also need to be kept informed as the evaluation proceeds, so they understand if there are concerns regarding their candidacy.

FUNCTIONAL CHARACTERISTICS

A social group for pre- and posttransplant cardiac patient operates at the level of a multifunctional group. There is a threefold functional focus: (1) education, (2) psychotherapy, and (3) support. The social group worker needs to have a complete understanding of how heart transplant works, its limitations, and the constraints (or limitations relative to cardiac patients who have been transplanted) involved in the process.

As a therapy group, the social group worker needs to help potential transplant patients discuss their concerns, worries, and fears. For posttransplant heart patients, the social group worker needs to help members accept responsibility for their ongoing care and address their trepidations, concerns, and fears. Moreover, the social group worker needs to help members understand their personal limitations at posttransplant.

Each social group for heart transplant patients has to provide a supportive environment for patients to share feelings, concerns, and fears, as well as the freedom to discuss barriers and obstacles, both interpersonal and medical. It is the responsibility of the social group worker to create this type of therapeutic environment.

Noncompliance appears to be relatively common after transplantation. Furthermore, compliance in most areas of the medical regimen worsens over the first year after the transplant, just as it does for most patients who begin new medical therapies. For example, up to 20 percent of heart transplant recipients and 50 percent of kidney transplant recipients have been found to be noncompliant with prescribed immunosuppressant medications during a given twelve-month period in the early posttransplant years (Hathaway et al. 1999).

Transplant teams' concerns are not limited to patients' compliance. The pattern of noncompliance and the tendency for noncompliance in a particular area (e.g., alcohol recidivism) to affect or lead to noncompliance in another area (e.g., not following the medication regimen) are also concerns. Unfortunately, there does not appear to be a particular "profile" of noncompliance after organ transplantation, so compliance and patterns of noncompliance must be evaluated on a case-by-case basis. The social group worker needs to be able to assess noncompliance indices on an onging basis, as well as skills in enhancing compliance using a cost-benefit self-assessment of outcome expectations.

STRUCTURAL CHARACTERISTICS

Given the potential therapeutic nature of mixing pre- and post-transplant cardiac patients, it is recommended that the group be open-ended with no restrictions placed on number of sessions attended. However, the cardiac transplant group needs to be held at least weekly at the same time and in the same setting. The clinical rationale for this structural aspect is that it provides predictability and consistency for cardiac patients who have grave concerns about the transplant process.

Numerous investigators have reported that important psychosocial issues arise during this time period. Common psychosocial issues for patients, which need to be addressed within the social group context relate to coping with physical changes and early complications such as acute graft rejection, enduring the psychological highs and lows that sometimes occur as side effects of immunosuppressive agents such as corticosteroids, managing a complex posttransplant regimen that encompasses: (1) multiple medications and dosing schedules, (2) monitoring vital signs, (3) exercise and dietary prescriptions, (4) regular follow-up medical evaluations and laboratory tests, and (5) lifestyle restrictions related to smoking, alcohol, and other potentially harmful substances. Other psychosocial issues for patients that need addressing are altering self-perceptions (transitioning from their roles as critically ill or dying patients and family caregivers to roles and lifestyles that are less illness-focused); psychological acceptance of the transplant and, for cadaver donation recipients, dealing with the fact that someone lost their life just when they regained theirs; and coping with financial and economic issues (cost of transplant surgery, hospital stay, and/or follow-up care and medications).

Given these concerns, patients and respective family members often are very focused on staying in close contact with the transplant team after they have returned home. The complexity of their medical regimen can be daunting. Gaps in knowledge about patients' recovery and health care needs usually surface during this time and can lead to increased anxiety and anger. Patients and family members alike can be dismayed that the relationship problems that existed before and/or during the period of critical illness and transplant surgery continue after they return home. Ironically, the stress of the waiting period can actually serve to temporarily hold relationships together.

Consequently, high levels of emotional distress, as well as clinically significant depression and anxiety-related disorders, are more frequent during the first posttransplant year than during later years for all types of organ transplantation. The occurrence of some psychiatric disorders such as transplant-related post-traumatic stress disorder (PTSD) may be limited almost exclusively to the first year after transplantation. Individuals with transplant-related PTSD appear to be unable to come to terms with the transplant experience and may experience flashbacks, nightmares, and extreme distress when thinking about or reminded of stressors during the waiting period, the surgery, and/or the recovery period. PTSD in transplant recipients has only recently received attention. There is also evidence that psychological problems during the first year influence physical health and well-being in subsequent years, further suggesting the need for early intervention.

GROUP LEADERSHIP SKILLS

The social group worker needs to help groups develop a sense of cohesion and support. The social group worker leading a group dealing with heart transplantation will need to develop skills and abilities in the following areas of clinical practice:

- Thorough, comprehensive understanding of the physiological aspects of how heart patients are referred for transplant
- How heart transplantation affects individuals physiologically and psychosocially
- An understanding of how individual's respond to potential life-threatening illnesses
- An understanding of and empathy for the effects of a heart transplantation on individual group members
- An understanding of how males versus females develop, cope, and manage heart transplantation
- Alternative ways for cardiac patients evaluated for heart transplant to utilize external resources
- An understanding of how family members deal with potentially life-threatening illness such as heart transplantation

Since not all heart transplants are successful, some resulting in death or protracted complications, the social group worker also needs to have skills in helping members deal with loss and death while continuing to instill hope for those who have been evaluated for transplant and those recently transplanted. If the social group worker is unable to respond to requested information, the worker needs to develop an appreciation and understanding of when and how to refer cardiac patients evaluated for heart transplant to other professionals who can address more medically technical concerns in a timely manner.

CLINICAL TECHNIQUES UTILIZED

The social group worker leading a cardiac transplant group needs to utilize an array of clinical skills. First, he or she needs to be able to impart technical information about the social aspects of heart transplant as well as have a good fundamental understanding of the medical complexities and procedural processes. Second, he or she needs to be able to utilize advanced group skills in an interactive process-oriented form. These techniques increase group cohesion, promote open communication of feelings, and provide a forum for understanding and empathy.

In keeping with the interpersonal nature of this approach, the primary focus of the group work is on the relationships among the group members and what is happening at the moment in the group. The group becomes a microcosm for members' lives, and any interpersonal problems they have will most likely occur sooner or later with someone in the group. Thus, rather than just talking about the problems in their lives (i.e., awaiting heart transplantation or having been recently transplanted), members act them out in the group, and this gives them a chance to get feedback on the way they impact others, to become aware of their feelings and motivations, and to experiment with new, healthier behaviors.

During this process, the leader facilitates the group members to help them increase awareness of what they are feeling in the moment, especially in response to what the other person just said, and help them to improve their communication skills, especially assertiveness and sensitivity to others. The leader is particularly interested in helping members to become aware of their interpersonal patterns, such as neediness, avoidance of intimacy, defiance of authority, and codependence. For each pattern, clients are helped to be aware of when it happens in the group, what they are feeling at the time, the underlying motivation, its childhood origin, and the role it plays in their lives. Then, they can work on healing the pain that underlies the pattern and experiment with healthier behavior in the group.

Other common types of group work involve encouraging cardiac patients to explore their feelings about being in the group, or the group-as-a-whole exploring an issue that is affecting everyone. The interpersonal work for each client changes over time. When people first join a group, they work on the way they relate to people they are just getting to know. Once they have been in the group for a period of time, they will have a chance to develop close connections with some other group members, and they will begin to deal with intimacy issues such as their inner fears relative to life and death.

Finally, the social group worker promotes members of a cardiac transplant group to develop a support system with other group members and the social group worker. For individuals faced with the decision of cardiac transplant, and those who have been transplanted, they need to feel that they are not alone. They need empathy, instillation of hope that their life can and will improve, and development of interpersonal learning (i.e., identification of maladaptive styles of adaptation and imitation of other group members' healthy interactions and approaches).

EXPECTED CLINICAL BENEFITS
AND OUTCOMES

The most important outcome for cardiac patients involved in a cardiac heart failure social group is that individual patients develop the following:

1. A basic understanding of how the heart transplant process works and the medical rationale for referral itself
2. Empowerment to be self-directed in treatment decisions and an openness to accept the outcomes of decisions made
3. An increase in feelings of self-mastery and hope gained through obtaining relevant information

4. An acceptance of the group support to enhance the cardiac patient's sense of connectedness through group cohesion and interpersonal involvement
5. Understanding the overall effects of how a cardiac patient, either referred for heart transplant or a recently transplanted patient, affects the family
6. An understanding of what the cardiac patient referred for transplantation, or recently transplanted, needs to do to be medically and psychosocially compliant
7. Through a basic understanding of the medical and psychosocial criteria for heart transplant, the cardiac patient will be able to make informed life and medical decisions
8. A willingness to accept support from group members
9. Development of a connectedness to an appropriate cardiac support group
10. Through a more comprehensive understanding of heart transplantation and the medical limitations, development of a lifestyle that minimizes organ rejection.

CONCLUSIONS

Heart transplantation is the most complicated cardiac intervention conducted. For the cardiac patient referred for transplantation, there is a natural fear factor present. Through the social group work process, candidates for heart transplant are able to interact with those who have gone before them and survived. This provides an instillation of hope during an extremely stressful decision making process and procedure. By gaining support and cogent information, the cardiac patient can make an informed decision and exercise his or her free will and self-determination.

Chapter 10

Stress Management Social Work Group for Cardiac Patients

INTRODUCTION

Historically, high blood pressure has been viewed as "a silent killer" in as much as individuals are often unaware of their blood pressure and are often equally unaware of the potential medical dangers associated with elevated blood pressure. Stress can be viewed as the other "silent killer," since many individuals are unaware of the level of stress they are under and generally do not understand the critical inverse connection between stress and health.

To live life is to experience stress in its many forms. But those who manage stress in healthy ways tend to lower their health risk factors in general, and specifically, stress management has been shown to help persons diagnosed with cardiovascular disease. Beyond biology and heredity, stress has been shown to worsen cardiac patients' condition and affective recovery rates. Developing psychosocial skills in the management of stress has been shown to improve the recovery rates for cardiac patients (Blumenthal et al. 1997, 1999).

RATIONALE FOR USING THE SOCIAL GROUP WORK MODEL

Behavioral theory argues that stress, not controlled by the individual, will manifest itself in a higher likelihood for irresponsible,

Social Group Work with Cardiac Patients
© 2007 by The Haworth Press, Inc. All rights reserved.
doi:10.1300/5739_10

inappropriate thoughts and behaviors in order to decrease negative feelings (depression, anxiety, worry, and so on). Keeping in mind that one can change thoughts and behaviors more easily than one can manipulate and change affective (feeling) components. Also, the association between cognitions, feelings, and behaviors does not occur in a vacuum; it is affected by social-environmental influences and one's genetic leaning (e.g., medical and biologic history on both biologic parents' family sides).

Stress can be defined as a circumstance in a person's life that causes tension or dysphoria. Stressors may be mild (e.g., termination of a friendship) or catastrophic (e.g., suicide of a spouse) (Kaplan and Sadock 2004). Yet, within the confines of this definition, there are many so-called pleasurable experiences that are also quite stressful (e.g., a marriage that is planned, a planned childbirth, a job promotion, etc.). This definition does not stress (no pun intended) that there are biological propensities that each of us have, and under the "right" amount of stress we may manage our stress relative to our biological leanings, social context, and psychological understanding of what relieves emotional pain.

Stress can be of two types: stress can be either positive (e.g., individuals awaiting the birth of a planned child) or negative (e.g., individuals dealing with a chronic disease, such as CVD). Both can promote change: one type motivates while the other type inhibits change. That is to say, there is *eustress* (stress that is present, but considered a motivation) and *stress* (stress that is negative and promotes unhealthy choices and decision making).

A historic model for conceptualizing stress is the Stress-Diathesis Model. This model has typically been utilized to understand stress, as it relates to thought disturbances, such as schizophrenia, but the model is useful, in my estimation, in conceptualizing stress and eustress, since our goal is to minimize the negative stress (stress) and enhance and promote the positive stress (eustress). Kaplan, Sadock, and Grebb (1994) have defined the Stress-Diathesis Model as follows:

> The model postulates that a person may have a specific vulnerability (diathesis) that, when acted on by some stressful environmental influence, allows the symptoms . . . [mental health

problems or substance use/abuse] . . . to develop. In the most general stress-diathesis model, the diathesis or the stress can be biological or environmental or both. The environmental component can be either biological (e.g., an infection) or psychological (e.g., a stressful family situation or the death of a close relative). The biological basis of a diathesis can be further shaped by epigenetic influences, such as substance abuse, psychological stress, and trauma. (pp. 606-608)

All humans react to stressful situations, whether real or imagined. The American Psychiatric Association (2000) considers a *stress reaction* to be a sudden, inadequate emotional reaction to a disastrous event or situation. These reactions may be chronic.

In addition, each person experiences a certain amount of stress on a daily basis, perhaps hour to hour. Each person will revert to his or her learned or biologically or culturally inherited reactions to the perceived stress. Some of this daily stress is motivational, such as test anxiety, which promotes a heightened sense of awareness through increased adrenaline. While other stressful situations can, and do, promote mental health problems from avoidance, to flight/fear, to one "freezing-up" to the point of making no change, either responsible or otherwise.

PURPOSE/GOALS

Many self-help books and programs claim, to varying degrees, to help stressed people minimize, reduce, or eradicate the stress in one's life. Yet, to make changes in stress management requires using alternative ways of thinking and behaving when stress begins to immobilize an individual. In essence, stress, whether positive or negative, needs to be managed; to not manage stress and find alternative ways to reduce the pressure is like allowing a pressure cooker to continually develop steam without a release valve.

There are several goals inherent in conducting social work groups that focus on stress control:

- Development of understanding what stress is and how it manifests itself in general and specifically related to cardiovascular disease
- Develop methods for identifying stressors of two types:
  —Positive stressors: those that tax the individual's physical and psychosocial self and emanate from overtly healthy sources (e.g., the birth of a planned child)
  —Negative stressors: those that tax the individual's physical and psychosocial self and emanate from overtly unhealthy sources (e.g., death of a loved one)
- Identifying and detecting major stressors in the cardiac patients life relative to the following:
  —Socialized ways in which the patient sees stressors historically
  —Medical situation
  —External (social) situations
  —Internal (psychological) constructions
  —Develop and hone healthy stress control and management techniques that best fit the individual's lifestyle

FUNCTIONAL CHARACTERISTICS

The social group model of stress control and management combines and integrates the following elements into a clear and comprehensive approach: established clinical theory about how individuals identify and manage stressors, empirically supported cognitive-behavioral clinical principles, and pragmatic clinical experience. The stress management social group combines both a forum for educating the cardiac patient and helping the client process ways to develop, hone, and utilize cognitive-behavioral techniques.

Gier, Levick, and Blazina (1988) were among the first to study stress reduction methods with cardiac patients and their families. They found that stress reduction methods, typically offered in social group formats, were demonstrated to show a positive effect, both empirically and qualitatively. The objective of this research program was to educate the participants in a variety of coping and stress reducing techniques to help prepare them for the multitude of stressors encountered during a major cardiac event or illness.

STRUCTURAL ASPECTS

Much of the material is provided using educational methods; that is, teaching clients how to recognize and identify stressors, detect underlying cognitive thoughts and perceptions that promote stress, challenge the underlying thoughts and perceptions, and developing behaviors that work to decrease and minimize stressors.

It is suggested that social work groups dealing with stress management meet at least weekly. Irrespective of the cardiac patient disease, it is helpful to have a heterogeneous mix relative to disease type and sex. Group membership should be between eight to ten cardiac patients to maximize the learning process on an individual basis as well as enhance interaction and discussion. Group sessions should be conducted at least weekly and cover the following areas of stress management:

Week 1: Understanding of Stress in General and Specifically Related to Cardiac Patients

Relationship Between Stress and Ongoing Cardiac Problem

- Addresses the correlations between cardiovascular disease and depression, anxiety, and anger
- Addresses the relationship of stress in concert with heredity and social lifestyle issues
- Understanding of what stress is (e.g., positive and negative stressors)
- Understanding the healthy aspects of stress for humans
- Understanding the critical connection between cognitions (thoughts and perceptions), behaviors (actions), and emotive (feeling/affect outcomes)

People can agree on ways to determine if stress is helpful or the destructive. Stress, by its nature, implies change; change in parts of the cardiac patient's life will result in some level or degree of stress. Imagined change, such as in "worry" and "guilt" cognitive constructs, is even stressful. Any situation that causes change in the cardiac patient's daily routine is stressful, whether positive or negative. Anything that causes change in the cardiac patient's health is stressful as well.

Whether or not the stress source is internal or external, positive or negative, individuals experience stress in as much the same manner. In its many forms, stress has an accrual effect. That is to say, whether stress is internal (e.g., worry or guilt) or external (e.g., the loss of a loved one or developing medical complications in an individual's illness).

Week 2: Highlighting the Difference Between Worry (Future-Oriented Thoughts/Perceptions) and Guilt (Historic-Oriented)

In delineating the differences between worry and guilt, it is important to help participants understand that these variables occur on a continuum. The group leader should emphasize that worry is a future-oriented process involving focus on potential negative outcomes that may or may not materialize. In comparison, guilt is a process in which the individual ruminates about past events in a manner that further compounds present life stressors.

Participants should be assisted toward understanding that worry and guilt are each manifestations of stress and are not dichotomous. An important therapeutic goal is recognition of the connection between stress level, emotional problems and substance use/abuse and mental illness (i.e., depression and anxiety). It is essential that the members are able to identify the sources of their personal stress, along with recognition of their individualized manifestations of stress in the "present moment." Moreover, understanding and appreciating the need for, and acceptance of, professional help is optimal.

In addressing the manifestations of stress, it is important to underscore that any situation that causes change in one's daily routine is stressful, whether positive or negative. Anything that causes change in an individual's health is stressful as well. Based on Burns and Burns (1990) seminal work in the area of stress identification, the following list represents a good fundamental understanding of how stress is manifested:

1. *Emotional stress:* Occurs when there are arguments, disagreements, and interpersonal conflicts that cause changes in an individual's personal life.

2. *Medical/physical illness:* Catching a cold, being infected with a virus, breaking an arm or leg, a skin lesion, a sore back are all changes in one's body condition.

3. *Pushing your body too hard:* A major source of stress is overdriving one's self. If an individual is working (or partying) sixteen hours daily, he or she will have reduced the available time for adequate rest. Sooner or later, the energy drain on the individual's system will cause the body to fall behind in its repair work. There will not be enough time or energy for the body to fix broken cells, or replace used brain cells. Change will occur in the body's internal environment. If one continues, permanent damage may be done. The body's fight to stay healthy in the face of the increased energy that one is expending is a major stress.

4. *Environmental factors:* Climate and other weather changes can be stressful. Very cold or very hot climates and very high altitudes can be stressful exposures to toxins, chemical or interpersonal, are stressful events. Each of these environmental factors serves to threaten a change in the body's internal environment.

5. *Allergic stress:* Allergic reactions are a part of an individual body's natural defense mechanism. When confronted with a substance that the human body considers toxic, the body will try to get rid of it, attack it, or somehow neutralize it. This applies to things that one breathes in or foreign objects one ingests, which assault an individual in a tactile way. Typically, medical doctors define an allergy as a definite stress, requiring large changes in energy expenditure on the part of a human body's defense system that has to fight off what the body perceives as a dangerous attack by an outside toxin.

6. *Hormonal stress factors:* Throughout one's life, myriad hormonal changes occur, which produce physical changes and ultimate stresses. For instance, puberty, premenstrual symptoms, and menopause create the vast majority of hormonal changes and are severe stressors. Here the body actually changes chemically, as hormones are released in large quantities.

7. *Taking responsibility for another's thoughts, behaviors, or feeling:* This responsibility is a major source of stress for both the person being controlled and the person taking on such a bur-

den. This is especially true for the cardiac patient that the only person he or she can control is himself or herself. Individuals never control other people; it's an illusion at best, and a delusion at worst.

Week 3: Strategies to Self-Manage Stress in Proactive, Prosocial Ways

- Understanding and using cognitive strategies
- Understanding and using behavioral strategies
- Enhancement of personal responsibility for the direction of and management of stress
- Assessing one's own limitations in cardiac recovery

It has been estimated that one in ten individuals are functioning in an overstressed mode at any given time throughout the day. This serves as an example that 10 percent of our citizens are immobilized by negative stress reactions, which affect their biological leanings, social situations, and psychological health. On the other hand, those with stress levels below the other nine people handle their stress, good or bad, in a responsible, appropriate manner.

Symptoms of overstress can range from depression, mania, anxiety attacks, substance use (licit or illicit), and compulsive behaviors, to gross refractory mental illness (thought disturbance) and substance use disorders (licit or illicit substance abuse or dependency).

The following techniques, derived from Burns and Burns (1990), gives practical, common sense actions for cardiac patients to take to help manage stress:

Make Life Predictable

Resetting one's body clock is vital if one is to feel well, sleep soundly, and wake refreshed. Give oneself a definite wake-up and sleep time. This sets a frame of reference for your body. Burns and Burns (1990) suggest that it may take several weeks to recalibrate one's body's normal sleep patterns.

Give Yourself a Break

An individual must give the human body adequate time to repair itself, and to regenerate the brain chemicals that produce a sense of control and tranquility in one's life. Overstress can result in fatigue, anger, aches and pains, problems with sleeping (falling to sleep and/ or staying asleep), lack of enjoyment in one's life, depression, and substance use (licit or illicit).

The recovering cardiac patient needs to allow the mind and body a chance to heal itself. Learning theory that undergirths cognitive-behavioral techniques suggests that, on average, it may take at least six months to get one back to "factory settings." A helpful cognitive-behavioral device is the use of the acronym GONE for organizing your life:

> Got to do: the three or four projects that need completion today
> Ought to do: those things that will become "Got to do's" tomorrow
> Nice to do: these are the follow-up activities that individuals like to do, such as write that late thank-you note, return a call to a friend who called several weeks ago, etc.
> Extras: these are all the extra things in one's life that he or she would like to do if only one had the time!

Lighten Your Load of Social Engagements

Let someone else place the holiday decorations on the Christmas tree. Use paper plates rather than the nice china. Go out only once a week. Tell visitors from out of town (who always expect to stay at the patient's house) to call "just as soon as they settle in a hotel room." Saying no is difficult, but can serve to help protect time and space.

Postpone Making Any Changes in Your Living Environment

Recall that change is stress. So relax and postpone any big moves for a while. Any change planned for the cardiac patient's living environment can be simultaneously exciting and stressful.

Reduce the Number of Hours Spent at Work or School

If one is an excessive worker, either in a job or in school, you need to reduce the energy drain placed on the body. Beyond forty hours of work or school-related activities weekly is unhealthy.

Eat More Healthy

People all vow to do this, but seldom do. Most individuals have learned the four basic food groups in school, but have gravitated to only one or two. If one eats only one "big" meal daily, it would be healthier and stress reducing to break that large meal into three smaller meals.

Stop Putting Yourself Down

Quit thinking of yourself in only negative terms. Give yourself the credit for the good things that one does on a daily basis—recall that people are not all good or all bad; people's behaviors are on a continuum.

Reduce the Pace of Your Life

Ask yourself, "Why am I in such a hurry? Where am I going and how fast do I need to go to get there?" Slow it down!

Get Some Basic Exercise

You must attempt on at least a thrice-weekly basis to invest in yourself. The typical American does everything else he or she wants to, except get a bit of exercise. Walking is a fully acceptable aerobic exercise and one that can also serve as a period of meditation.

Set Priorities

Decide what is most important, and do it first.

Learn to Say No and Mean It

Being asked to do something above and beyond what an individual has to do (see the GONE method, mentioned earlier) is often a compliment, but if accepting the task is going to add undue stress to one's life, then gracefully say, "No."

Take Time to Think Before Acting

If you are starting a new project, think about how best to tackle it before beginning. If you are running errands around town, plan the trip so as to not waste time retracing your steps.

Make Lists to Organize Your Work, Thoughts, and Time

Before phoning someone or going into a meeting, make a list of the points you want to discuss, and prioritize them with numbers. That way, you will be sure to cover the most important event if time runs short.

Finish One Task Before Starting Another

You will not waste time redoing tasks that were misunderstood, or feel frustrated when someone else responds in a manner you think they should not.

Listen Carefully

Get the facts right upfront. An individual will not waste time redoing tasks that were misunderstood, or feel frustrated when someone else responds in a way the person thinks they should not have.

Finish the Most Important Tasks First

One may think they are accomplishing a lot if one just start "doing something," but an individual may run out of time and leave the most important items (in their estimation) incomplete.

Do Not Dwell on the Past

The past is history—one cannot change it. The present is in your control, and the future has not arrived. Practice "present moment living."

Do Not Dwell on the Future

This is a form of worry. Always plan carefully, but accept that you cannot influence or control the future.

Concentrate on Creating a Success

Stop spending time on unproductive activities. If you are "spinning" your wheels in an "emotional snowbank," stop, get on the cell phone, and call for help. Focus on the tasks that truly accomplish something.

Stay in the Present Moment

This is the only moment an individual actually owns; use the time wisely.

Taking Responsibility for Another's Thoughts, Behaviors, or Feeling

Taking responsibility for another person's thoughts, behaviors, and/or feeling is a major source of stress for both the person being controlled and the person taking on such a burden. Remember that the only person you can control is yourself—individuals never control other people; as previously stated, it's an illusion at best, and a delusion at worst.

Week 4: The Role of Psychosocial Support in Cardiac Recovery

- Setting healthy boundaries with family members
- Including significant others and significant family members in the cardiac recovery process
- Appreciation for ongoing psychosocial support and commitment to cardiac recovery—lifestyle changes

Although most often difficult in the best of times, setting healthy boundaries is extremely important. Even though a cardiac patient may appear overtly to be quite well, individuals heal quicker on the outside than on the inside, both physically and psychosocially. Hence, the cardiac patient needs to be able to set healthy boundaries for himself or herself as well as for significant others, peers, co-workers, and supervisors.

GROUP LEADERSHIP SKILLS

Social workers conducting stress management groups need to have an excellent grasp of cognitive-behavioral techniques, such as cognitive challenges of irrational and erroneous thoughts, reframing of negative thoughts and worldviews, restructuring negative perceptions that underlie negative feelings, and stress. The social group worker needs to develop skills in helping cardiac patients improve social judgment and decision making by focusing on realistic outcome expectations. The social group worker should develop skills in helping cardiac patients plan to manage stress in the worse case scenario. The social group workers leading stress management groups need to develop a comfort zone for being able to create in vivo examples, as well as being able to use various metaphors and similes to enable cardiac patients to contemplate real-life stressful situations and alternative ways to respond to these stressors. Social group workers need to be able to help the cardiac group member identify current stressors and use the group process to generate possible and feasible alternative ways to address stressful situations.

CLINICAL TECHNIQUES UTILIZED

The social group worker will serve the role of trainer and process facilitator in a social group focused on stress management. It is important for the social group worker to normalize human stress, both positive and negative. Moreover, the social group worker will need to underscore that stress is implicit in human life, but that stress has an accrual effect (i.e., stress, whether positive or negative, can escalate).

Therefore, the cardiac patient will need to develop healthy alternatives to manage the stress.

Cognitive-behavioral techniques are utilized to help cardiac patients identify negative feelings (i.e., depression, stress, and anger); detect underlying negative or irrational thoughts; and actively challenge and reframe negative thoughts and restructure negative perceptions that underlie negative feelings and stressors. It is suggested that, as stress management material is presented, the social group helps the individual cardiac patient integrate various techniques into their psychosocial repertoire. Role-play is often utilized to allow cardiac patients to practice stress management skill development and refinement as the social group worker and fellow group members offer feedback and negative critique. Guided imagery is often used to help the cardiac patient mentally visualize stressful situations, be able to label the severity of the stressful situation, and cognitively practice alternative methods to intervene in healthy ways.

EXPECTED CLINICAL BENEFITS AND OUTCOMES

One of the most fundamental outcomes for cardiac patients involved in stress management social group work is that clients participate in developing an understanding of how stress affects individuals, both positive and negative. The cardiac patient will be able to articulate the effects of both positive and negative stress. He or she will have a more complete understanding of the triggers that promote stress and will be able to understand the negative thoughts and perceptions that promote stress. Also, the cardiac patient will be able to self-assess how stress affects them on an individual basis.

CONCLUSIONS

By participating in a cognitive-behavioral model of stress management, cardiac group members will be able to understand and utilize healthier alternative methods to manage stress in responsible and healthy ways. Historically, journalists have utilized their adage of "if one can frame it, one can claim it" to enhance their sense of mastery writing a byline or story. Put in stress-management terms, if one can identify stressors, one can learn to control them. Within the social group work context, cardiac patients learn how to identify stressors, both positive and negative, and utilize skills to manage stress in healthier ways. Thus, social group affords the cardiac patient the context in which to practice stress management and reduction techniques through cognitive-behavioral skill development, role-plays, and process element.

Chapter 11

Social Group Management
of Anger Among Cardiac Patients

INTRODUCTION

It has been said that anger corrodes the container in which it is held. Although anger is one of myriad human emotions, historically, unmanaged expressed anger and concealed anger has been thought to be detrimental to one's overall health physically, socially, and psychologically. Most observers of human emotions recognize that certain circumstances and actions by others seem to trigger anger responses. When one is intentionally hurt, insulted, cheated, deceived, or made fun of, it may arouse anger and possible aggression (Byrne and Kelley 1981). In most situations, humans perceive that others should treat them with consideration, fairness, and understanding; when these are not realized (i.e., reality of interpersonal situation falls short of our perceptions), people experience frustration. This frustration often is expressed behaviorally in anger. Thus, frustration leads to anger and possible aggression. The functional aspect of expressed anger keeps individuals at some social distance.

When an individual is diagnosed with a potentially life-threatening diagnosis, such as cardiac disease, the patient begins a psychosocial struggle and process to make sense of the illness. Elizabeth Kubler-Ross (1969, 1972, 1997) developed a model of personal change after spending time on analyzing the emotional responses to grief by terminally ill patients that is equally relevant to individuals diagnosed with a cardiac disease. The model identifies the human emotional response to change over time, which includes denial, anger, bargaining,

Social Group Work with Cardiac Patients
© 2007 by The Haworth Press, Inc. All rights reserved.
doi:10.1300/5739_11

depression, and acceptance. Although this model of change is not linear, after accepting the reality of having a cardiac disease, anger may become more predominate.

Anger can be defined as an emotional state that varies in intensity from irritation to intense fury and rage. Similar to other human emotions, anger is typically accompanied by physiological, biological, and psychosocial changes. At its core, anger is an emotion that raises heart rate and blood pressure, and requires increased energy for hormones such as adrenaline and noradrenaline. At the psychosocial level, anger tends to keep others away, which increases social and psychological isolation (Ludwig and Farrelly 1967).

Either external or internal events, or both, can trigger anger. One can be directed at a specific person or groups of people who perceptually have done something to trigger the response. Moreover, anger can be caused by worry (dwelling on what may or may not occur in the future), guilt (dwelling on what one could, should, or ought to have handled differently). In addition, traumatic or enraging events can also trigger an anger response.

The instinctual, natural way to express anger is to respond with aggression. Anger is a natural, adaptive response to perceived or real threats to one's safety. Anger inspires powerful, often aggressive feelings and behaviors that allow people to fight to defend themselves when attacked. Thus, a certain amount of anger is intrinsic to human survival.

On the other hand, people cannot physically lash out at every person or object that irritates or annoys them. Social norms, social conventions, laws, and common sense place limits on how far one's anger can be expressed. Therefore, whether anger is expressed or not, there is an accrual effect. That is to say, anger, similar to stress, builds up in one's psyche as well as one's physical health. Unless a person has a healthy way to dispense of anger, it continues to build to the point of aggressive outburst.

RATIONALE FOR USING
THE SOCIAL GROUP WORK MODEL

There is a correlation between anger and the incidence of cardiac stress (Chang et al. 2002). In general terms, numerous studies have proffered the negative connection between anger and the development or exacerbation of health problems. Developing anger management and control techniques improved ones overall sense of psychosocial stability (Deffenbacher 1995). Mismanaged anger has been shown to increase peoples' risk for numerous health problems (Deffenbacher 1995). Anger has also been shown to be associated with other behaviors that negatively affect health. For instance, in a study reported in *Cognitive Brain Research* (Fallon et al. 2004), it was shown that people with hostile aggressive personality traits are more likely to become addicted to nicotine, which has long been associated with increased risk for chronic health problems.

A small but critical and growing number of epidemiological studies have suggested that anger and hostility are related to incidence of cardiac disease (Mercola 2000; Thomas 1989; Williams et al. 2000). Tsaih and colleagues (2004) analyzed data from the Normative Aging Study that suggested higher levels of expressed anger are a risk factor for development of cardiac disease and that expressed anger may well worsen cardiac outcomes.

More recently, Dr. Chang and colleagues (2002) of the Johns Hopkins University School of Medicine studied a group of 1,000 men aged thirty-two years to forty-eight years and examined their incidence of premature heart disease compared with anger responses to stress during early adult life. Men who were classified as having the highest levels of anger reported experiencing expressed or concealed anger and irritability and were more than three times as likely to develop premature heart disease when compared with their less angry colleagues. Furthermore, those defined as having high rates of anger were more than six times more likely to have a heart attack by the age of fifty-five years.

PURPOSE/GOALS

The overriding purpose of conducting an anger management social work group with cardiac patients is to deal with four crucial dynamics. First, social group members need to normalize anger as a human emotion that has either positive or negative effects, irrespective of the myriad self-help books on the topic of anger in which anger is viewed a "bad emotion" that needs to be eradicated. However, anger, like all other human emotions, cannot be eliminated. That is to say, anger, as other emotions such as love, are part of the full complement of human emotions. One cannot eliminate anger anymore than one can eradicate feelings of love. The point is that having anger is human; understanding one's anger allows the patient to control it rather than vice versa. Second, patients need to identify, accept, and address that anger is a natural response to being evaluated and diagnosed with a chronic disease, such as cardiac disease. Third, the cardiac patient needs to appreciate that untreated and undirected anger may have contributed to the cardiac disease, as well as serving to exacerbate the disease itself. And, finally, the cardiac patient will need to move beyond anger in order to move into a recovery mode of acceptance.

FUNCTIONAL CHARACTERISTICS

A social group focused on anger management and control has to be didactic, experiential, and process-oriented. It is didactic in regard to imparting and teaching techniques that have a proven outcome. The group is experiential in the sense of helping cardiac patients make critical connections between an understanding and comprehension of anger as a human trait that has both positive and negative potential outcomes. The social group is process-oriented by allowing cardiac patients to grapple with alternative methods to integrate anger control in their lives. Uncontrolled anger can move to aggression and ultimately rage.

From a learning theory perspective that informs cognitive-behavior, it is denied that humans are innately aggressive and that frustration always leads to aggression. Instead, Bandura (1973) argues that aggression is learned in two fundamental ways: (1) from observing aggressive models and (2) from receiving and/or expecting payoffs following aggression. The payoffs or positive reinforcements may be in the form of stopping aggression in others, getting praise or status or some other goal by being aggressive, getting self-reinforcement and private praise, and/or reducing internal and biologic tension. From the learning theory perspective, the interpersonal and cognitive processes, such as rational problem solving, therapeutic rehearsals (role- plays that portray real-life situations), and self-control procedures of self-observation, self-evaluation, and self-reinforcement are all techniques that are utilized in management.

STRUCTURAL CHARACTERISTICS

The general material provided is based on educational methods; that is, teaching clients how to recognize and identify anger, detect underlying cognitive thoughts and perceptions that promote an anger response, challenge the underlying thoughts and perceptions that promote an anger response, and develop behaviors that work to minimize anger responses.

In addition, the social group worker needs to normalize anger as a natural response, especially when confronted with a major medical malady such as cardiovascular disease. The inherent issue is not that people need to eradicate anger, but need to make their anger work for them. An example typically utilized is to conceptualize anger as if one has an understanding of atomic energy. With an understanding of atomic energy, as with anger, once acknowledged, one can either make power or destroy things. The social group worker needs to normalize anger, not make anger a pathological condition.

It is suggested that social work groups dealing with anger management meet at least weekly. Irrespective of the cardiac patient disease, it is helpful to have a heterogeneous mix relative to disease type and sex. Group sessions should be conducted at least weekly and cover the following specific areas of stress management and control. Group size should be limited (e.g., eight to ten patient members) to enhance interaction and allow for individual attentions.

In addition, clients need to be able to discern the difference between anger and other emotions. If one can isolate and identify anger from other emotions, then one can affect a change. There is a traditional conceptualization by journalists: if one can frame it, one can claim it! Said differently, if you can identify and label anger, then one can take control of it, rather than anger controlling the patient.

The cardiac patient needs help and direction to appreciate that untreated and undirected anger may have contributed to the cardiac disease. Moreover, the cardiac patient needs to understand that unbridled anger may serve to exacerbate the disease itself. Finally, the cardiac patient needs help and guidance to move beyond anger, so as to appreciate negative effects that uncontrolled anger has a negative effect on cardiovascular recovery.

GROUP LEADERSHIP SKILLS

Beyond a working understanding of group dynamics, the social group worker needs to be able to facilitate processing of information and help the cardiac patient determine alternative methods to integrate these skills into their social context and within the patient's intrapsychic components.

The social group worker leading an anger management group must have the following skill sets. First, a worker must have a complete understanding of the management of anger and how anger manifests itself, especially in the midst of a chronic health problem such as cardiovascular disease. The social group worker needs to have a working and pragmatic understanding of anger and alternative methods to manage anger, as well as a complete understanding of cognitive-behavioral interventive models, especially relative to identifying anger. A worker should know how to detect the underlying negative thoughts and perceptions, and challenge and reframe negative thoughts, and restructure the underlying negative perceptions. The group worker needs also to be able to help the cardiac patient refine prosocial, proactive ways to solve interpersonal and social problems by actively challenging the outcome expectations for the cardiac patient and his or her family and significant others.

CLINICAL TECHNIQUES UTILIZED

Given the complex nature of anger relative to how it is triggered and its varying effects on individuals, the techniques need to be based on informed eclecticism. That is to say, no one method for managing anger is effective for all individuals. And in the final analysis, each individual who is able to recognize anger as a problem has to develop an individualized management methods. The following clinical techniques are suggested.

Relaxation

Simple relaxation tools such as deep breathing and relaxing imagery can help calm angry feelings. Some simple steps that can be recommended include teaching breathing techniques such as deep breathing from the diaphragm, since breathing from the chest does not tend to relax individuals. Have the patient picture his or her breath as coming up from the "gut," have the patient slowly repeat a calm word or phrase such as "relax," or "take it easy," and have the patient repeat it while breathing deeply.

Use imagery by having the patient visualize a relaxing experience, either from a positive memory or from one's imagination. Suggest using nonstrenuous, slow, yoga-like exercises that relax muscles and make the patient feel much calmer. The social group worker should promote daily patient practice of these techniques. This will help the patient learn to use them automatically during tense situations.

Cognitive Restructuring

Simply put, this means helping the cardiac patient change the way he or she thinks. Angry people tend to curse, swear, or speak in highly colorful terms that reflect their inner thoughts. When an individual is angry, thinking can get exaggerated and overly dramatic. Encourage the patient to try replacing these thoughts with more rational ones. For instance, instead of telling oneself, "oh, it's awful, it's terrible, everything's ruined," have the patient challenge these thoughts, "it's frustrating, and it's understandable that I'm upset about it, but it's not the end of the world, and getting angry is not going to fix it anyhow."

Caution the cardiac patient to be selective of words such as "never" or "always" when talking about one's self or someone else. Negative thoughts often serve to justify anger. These self-defeating thoughts also alienate and humiliate people who might otherwise be willing to work with the patient on a solution. The social group worker needs to underscore for the patient that getting angry is not going to fix anything, and that it won't make the individual feel better (and may actually make them feel worse).

Logic defeats anger because anger, even when it is justified, can quickly become irrational. Hence, suggest that the patient use cold, hard logic on himself or herself. Remind the patient that the world is not "out to get" him or her, instead underscore to the patient that he or she is experiencing some of the rough spots of daily life. As the cardiac patient practices challenging irrational thoughts, perception, and outcome expectation, this will lead to a more balanced perspective. Angry people tend to make demands: fairness, appreciation, agreement, and willingness to do things their way. Everyone wants these things, and they are all hurt and disappointed when they do not get them, but angry people *demand* them, and when their demands are not met, their disappointment becomes anger. As part of their cognitive restructuring, angry people need to become aware of their demanding nature and translate their expectations into desires. In other words, saying, "I would like" something is healthier than saying, "I demand" or "I must have" something. When one is unable to get what he or she wants, an individual will experience the normal reactions—frustration, disappointment, hurt—but not anger. Some angry people use this anger as a way to avoid feeling hurt, but highlight for the patient that anger doesn't mean the hurt goes away.

Problem Solving

Sometimes, anger and frustration are caused by very real and inescapable problems in our lives. Not all anger is misplaced, and often it's a healthy, natural response to these difficulties. There is also a cultural belief that every problem has a solution, and this adds to an individual's frustration to find out that this isn't always the case. It is noteworthy that not all perceived problems are solvable. This awareness is particularly upsetting to individuals who are either perfectionists in their worldview or who endeavor to use logic. Logic is not always helpful in solving problems, which are interpersonal in nature. The best attitude to bring to such a situation, then, is not to focus on finding the solution, but rather is helping the cardiac patient develop and explore alterative ways to face the problem. For example, help the patient to learn how to partialize a problematic situation or use a stepwise method in dividing a problem into more manageable steps. Also, help the patient use present moment thinking rather that dwelling in the past (i.e., use of guilt) or the future (i.e., worry).

Help the patient make manageable plans, and encourage them to check their progress along the way. Help the patient resolve to give it his or her best, but avoid punishing oneself if no answer is forthcoming. If the patient can approach problems with his or her best intentions and efforts and make a serious attempt to face it head-on, the individual will be less likely to lose patience and fall into "all-or-nothing thinking," even if the problem does not get solved right away. Finally, helping the patient challenge his or her outcome expectations (as in there being one way to solve a problem), can reduce the risks of increasing frustrations. The concept of equal-finality helps individuals understand that there are often multiple ways to get to the resolution of a complex problem.

Enhanced Communication

Angry people tend to react to, and act upon, perceptions and conclusions, and some of those conclusions can be very inaccurate. The first thing to do if one is in a heated discussion is slow down and think through your responses. Don't say the first thing that comes into your head, but slow down, and think carefully about what you want to say. At the same time, listen carefully to what the other person is saying and take your time before answering. This is the same principle that athletes use during the final stages of a sporting game: slow down and think about the next play; don't go in to the game and throw the ball wildly.

Encourage the cardiac patient to listen to what is underlying the anger. For instance, most individuals need to embrace a certain amount of freedom and personal space, and one's "significant other" wants more connection and closeness. If he or she starts complaining about the cardiac activities, promote the cardiac patient to not retaliate by painting his or her partner as a jailer, a warden, or an albatross around their neck.

It is natural to get defensive when one is criticized (this creates cognitive dissonance), but encourage the cardiac patient not to fight back (Festinger 1956). Instead, encourage the patient to listen to what is underlying the words: the message that this person might feel neglected and unloved. It may take a lot of cardiac patient's self-questioning to challenge his or her role in anger.

Using Humor

"Silly humor" can help defuse rage in a number of ways. For one thing, it can help one get a more balanced perspective. When a person gets angry and calls someone a name or refers to him or her in some imaginative phrase, have the patient stop and picture what that word would literally look like. If an individual is at work and thinks of a co-worker as a "dirtbag" or a "single-cell life form," for example, promote a cognitive picture of a large bag full of dirt (or an amoeba) sitting at your colleague's desk, talking on the phone, going to meetings. Do this whenever a name comes into your head about another person. If one can, draw a picture of what the actual thing might look like. This will take a lot of the edge off one's fury, and humor can always be relied upon to help unknot a tense situation.

The underlying message of highly angry people, Dr. Deffenbacher (1995) notes, that these people tend to feel that they are morally right, that any blocking or changing of their plans is an unbearable indignity and that they should not have to suffer this way. Maybe other people do, but not them!

When one feels this urge, the social group worker can suggest a picture of the cardiac patient as a god or goddess, a supreme ruler, who owns the streets and stores and office space, striding alone and having their way in all situations, while others defer to them. The more detail one can get into his or her imaginary scenes, the more chances one has to realize that maybe he or she is being unreasonable; the cardiac patient can also realize how unimportant the things they are angry about really are.

There are two cautions in using humor. First, do not try to have the cardiac patient just "laugh off" his or her problems; rather, use humor to help the patient face them more constructively. Second, encourage the cardiac patient to not give in to harsh, sarcastic humor; that is just another form of unhealthy anger expression.

What these techniques have in common is a refusal to take oneself too seriously. Anger is a serious emotion, but it is often accompanied by ideas that, if examined, can make an individual laugh.

Changing One's Environment

Sometimes an individual's immediate surroundings can trigger them to irritation and fury. Problems and responsibilities can weigh on individuals and make them feel angry at the "trap" he or she seems to have fallen into and all the people and things that form that trap. Encourage the cardiac patient to give himself or herself a break. Ensure that the cardiac patient has some "personal time" scheduled for times of the day that he or she knows are particularly stressful.

The following are ancillary environmental strategies for helping the cardiac patient to manage anger:

- *Timing:* If the cardiac patient and his or her partner tend to fight when discussing things at night—perhaps the individual is tired, or distracted, or maybe it's just habit—suggest changing the times when one talks about important matters so these talks don't turn into arguments.
- *Avoidance:* If the patient's child's chaotic room makes the patient furious every time he or she walks by it, shut the door. Tell them, "Don't make yourself look at what infuriates you. Don't say, 'Well, my child should clean up the room so I won't have to be angry!' That's not the point. The point is to keep yourself calm."
- *Finding alternatives:* If the patient's daily commute through traffic leaves the individual in a state of rage and frustration, suggest a project—learning or maping out a different route, one that's less congested or more scenic. Or finding another alternative, such as a bus or commuter train.

EXPECTED CLINICAL BENEFITS AND OUTCOMES

Anger is particularly destructive in relationships. When we live in close contact with someone, our personalities, priorities, interests, and ways of doing things frequently clash. Since we spend so much time together, and since we know the other person's shortcomings so well, it is very easy for us to become critical and short-tempered with our partner and to blame him or her for making our life uncomfortable.

Unless we make a continuous effort to deal with this anger as it arises, our relationship will suffer. Anger and the management thereof is particularly complex when a family member is dealing with major medical crises, such as cardiovascular illness.

In reality, most emotional problems are nothing more than a failure to accept things as they are, or an attempt to control and/or manipulate the psychosocial environment—in which case, it is patient acceptance, rather than attempting to change externals, that is the solution. For example, many of our relationship problems arise because individuals do not accept their partner as he or she is. In these cases, the solution is not to change our partner into what we would like him or her to be, but to accept them fully as they are. There are many levels of acceptance.

Through the development of anger management and controls, allow the cardiac patient to develop acceptance of others. Once the cardiac patients fully accepts other people as they are, without the slightest judgment or critique—as all the enlightened beings accept us—then, there is no basis for problems in the individual's relations with others. Problems do not exist outside our mind, so when the cardiac patient stops seeing other people as problems, they stop being problems. A core principle of anger control is that individuals cannot change other people in their social context; an individual can only change how he or she responds to others.

Patient acceptance not only helps the cardiac patient, it also helps those people with whom the individual interacts. Being accepted feels very different to being judged. When someone feels judged, they automatically become tight and defensive, but when they feel accepted, they can relax, and this allows their good qualities to come to the surface.

Finally, as the cardiac patient develops skills in anger control, this will have several positive effects, such as reduction of internal negative stressors, which negatively affect one's cardiac condition (e.g., more stable blood pressure); promotion of personal responsibility for one's reactions to others in both psychosocial and environmental contexts; decrease in the overall judgment of significant others in the patient's life; and create an inverse effect, by pulling significant people emotionally closer, especially during a period of chronic cardiac disease.

CONCLUSIONS

Once educated about anger and empowered to act appropriately on behalf of his or her rights as a human being, each cardiac patient has a vital obligation to assess his or her impact on others. Each has a part to play in creating a more humane and satisfying workplace, and ultimately, a more powerful profession. Anger and conflict will always be present in the stressful health care environment. However, intelligent management is possible—and indeed, urgently needed. Through the use of social groups, cardiac patients are able to gain an understanding of anger, how it affects the patient, and his or her family, as well as learning alternative ways to express anger. Finally, by proactively managing one's stressors, this will minimize the risks of additional cardiovascular disease.

Chapter 12

Cardiac Patient
Substance Abuse Group

INTRODUCTION

With the recognition that addiction, in its many forms, permeates most forms of clinical practice irrespective of treatment setting as well as most major medical problems, the demand for concise evaluation and treatment for substance use has increased. Social group work and addiction treatment are natural allies. This is partly because individuals who abuse substances are more often willing to stay sober and committed to treatment when it is provided in social groups, apparently because of the rewarding and therapeutic benefits such as affiliation, confrontation, support, gratification, and identification. The overall capacity of social group work to bond individuals having a substance use disorder to treatment is an important asset because greater the amount, quality, and duration of treatment, the better the patient's prognosis.

With the evaluation of cardiac patients, the first major step is to rule out any historic or current substance use disorders in the form of misuse, abuse, or dependency. After assessing the presence of substance use, the next step is to determine the severity of substance abuse or dependency. Finally, the social group worker needs to assess the relative motivation of the cardiac patient who has a substance use disorder as to his or her willingness to clinically address this problem.

Social Group Work with Cardiac Patients
© 2007 by The Haworth Press, Inc. All rights reserved.
doi:10.1300/5739_12

RATIONALE FOR USING
THE SOCIAL GROUP WORK MODEL

The majority of patients admitted for cardiovascular disease have no history of substance abuse or dependency. However, there are some who have exhibited abuse (a judgment problem) and dependency (either a physical and/or psychological addiction). The most common legal (for individuals aged eighteen years and above in most states) drugs that cardiac patients present with are nicotine (e.g., snuff, cigarettes, chewing tobacco), caffeine, and alcohol. There are more limited number of cardiac patients who have had a history of illicit substance abuse (e.g., cocaine, heroin, THC [cannabis], hallucinations, and methamphetamines). In addition, many of the cardiac patients admitted for heart care have used multiple substances within hours of a major cardiac event.

MOST PROBLEMATIC DRUGS
FOR CARDIAC PATIENTS

The core licit and illicit drugs that typically present the greatest challenge for the cardiac patients are as follows:

Nicotine

Nicotine is an agonist of the acetylcholine receptor; it is also the most prevalent psychoactive drug in the world. Nicotine is the main component of tobacco, which is used to make cigarettes, cigars, and smokeless tobacco, or snuff. Although there are many other compounds that are found in cigarettes, nicotine is the chemical that is responsible for their addictive nature. Approximately 35 million Americans smoke as a result of the addictive properties of nicotine. There are many new treatments available to help stop this deadly addiction, but research has shown that unless these smokers are willing to quit, these therapies are not extremely effective (Kannel 1978).

The effects of nicotine and smoking are extremely dangerous and often deadly. Smoking can produce a rapid addiction to nicotine that can last for a lifetime. Although there are many forms of treatment available to fight this powerful addiction, the success rate for most of these products is quite low. Group counseling, as well as a combination of available products, seems to be the most successful form of treatment. However, the primary reason these therapies often fail is the individual's lack of will and determination. Most studies conducted have determined that these treatments are not as effective unless the individual is motivated to stop their addiction. Smoking can lead to cardiovascular disease, lung disease, cancer, and birth defects, among many other things (Garrison, Feinleib, Castelli, and McNamara 1983). Smokers must realize that their addiction causes harm not only to themselves, but also to the people around them.

Caffeine

Some individuals just cannot get through a morning or even a day without caffeine. Many studies have been done about caffeine, but the results and conclusions tend to vary, contradict, or change as technology evolves.

Caffeine is known in the medical world as trimethylxanthine. It can be used medically as a cardiac stimulant or as a diuretic. Some studies seem to say that caffeine acts like drugs such as amphetamines, cocaine, or nicotine. These studies suggest that caffeine affects the part of the brain that triggers functional activity in the shell of the nucleus accumbens (the part of the brain responsible for addiction). This seems to be old news. Researchers have discovered that caffeine does not affect the area of the brain that involves addiction at doses of one to three cups a day (Corti, Binggeli, and Sudano 2002). One to three cups will increase alertness, but will not fulfill the addictive dependence.

The amount of caffeine present in one's cup of coffee depends on many variables. Drip coffee has about 100 mg of caffeine in a six-ounce cup. A double shot of espresso has about 50 mg of caffeine.

For a period of time, it was thought that caffeine contributed to heart disease, high blood pressure, miscarriage, and many other medical problems. Recently, with more rigorous testing and better methods, the American Medical Association stated that moderate tea or coffee drinkers probably need not have concern for their health relative to their caffeine consumption, provided other lifestyle habits (diet, alcohol consumption) are moderate, as well (Winkelmayer 2005). Of all the studies done so far, there has been no evidence that serious health problems occur as a result of drinking coffee or having caffeine in your diet. It is recommended that your caffeine intake is not more than 300 mg per day. That's about three cups of drip-brewed coffee per day. For those individuals who drink beyond 300 mg per day, the chance of developing medical problems increases (Kim 2003).

Stress, coffee, and caffeine increase the incidence of heart palpitations, cardiac arrhythmias, and homocystine, which are all risk factors for heart disease. Research suggests that more the coffee consumed (over 300 mg per day), the greater the risk of heart attack (Kim 2003).

Coffee and caffeine increase levels of the stress hormone called cortisol. Both coffee and caffeine elevate cortisol, and drinking regular and decaf coffee have all been shown to significantly increase systolic and diastolic blood pressure. High blood pressure is one of the most significant risk factors for heart disease. One can lower his or her stress levels by quitting coffee and caffeine intake.

Coffee and caffeine intake aggravate stress, including physical, mental, and emotional, by increasing the production of the stress hormone called cortisol. Increased levels of cortisol are associated with insulin resistance, fat cravings, and increased appetite. In addition, elevated cortisol creates fat deposits on the abdomen. Caffeine consumption also increases the tendency of people to overeat or binge eat, causing weight gain. Quitting caffeine can help people get a handle on emotional eating and weight gain by reducing the stress hormone cortisol.

An individual's immune system is weakened when stress hormones are chronically elevated. This accelerates a number of disease processes, including cardiovascular disease and immune system dysfunction. It's hard enough to get a handle on our daily stress without unnecessarily contributing to it. Quitting that coffee habit can be an important step toward reducing an individual's risk of disease (Winkelmayer 2005).

Alcohol

Excessive alcohol can raise the levels of some fats in the blood (triglycerides). It can also lead to high blood pressure, heart failure, and an increased calorie intake. (Consuming too many calories can lead to obesity and a higher risk of developing diabetes.) Excessive drinking and binge drinking can also lead to stroke. Other serious problems include fetal alcohol syndrome, cardiomyopathy cardiac arrhythmia, and sudden cardiac death (Lucas, Ledgerwood, and Kline 2000).

It is suggested that if you must drink alcohol, do so in moderation. This means, an average of one to two drinks per day for men and one drink per day for women. (A drink is one 12 oz. beer, 4 oz. of wine, 1.5 oz. of 80-proof spirits, or 1 oz. of 100-proof spirits.) Drinking more alcohol increases dangers such as alcoholism, high blood pressure, obesity, stroke, breast cancer, suicide, and accidents (CDC 1983; Waller 1972). Also, it's not possible to predict in which people alcoholism will become a problem. In view of these facts and other risks, the American Heart Association cautions people *not* to start drinking alcohol if the patient does not already do so (AHA 1998).

Over the past several decades, many studies have been published in science journals about how drinking alcohol may be associated with reduced mortality due to heart disease in some populations. Some researchers have suggested that the benefit may be due to wine, especially red wine. Others are examining the potential benefits of components in red wine such as flavonoids and other antioxidants in reducing heart disease risk. Some of these components may be found in other foods such as grapes or red grape juice. The linkage reported in many of these studies may be due to other lifestyle factors rather than alcohol. Such factors may include increased physical activity, and a diet rich in fruits and vegetables and lower in saturated fats. No direct comparison trials have been done to determine the specific effect of wine or other alcohol on the risk of developing heart disease or stroke.

The best-known effect of alcohol is a small increase in HDL cholesterol. However, regular physical activity is another effective way to raise HDL cholesterol, and niacin can be prescribed to raise it to a greater degree. Alcohol or some substances such as resveratrol found in alcoholic beverages may prevent platelets in the blood from sticking together. This may reduce clot formation and thus, reduce the risk of heart attack or stroke. (Aspirin may help reduce blood clotting in a similar way.) How alcohol or wine affects cardiovascular risk merits further research, but right now the American Heart Association does not recommend drinking wine or any other form of alcohol to gain these potential benefits (AHA 1998). However, the AHA recommends that to reduce one's risk, an individual should talk to a doctor about lowering cholesterol and blood pressure, controlling your weight, getting enough exercise, and following a healthy diet (AHA 1998, 2005b). There is no scientific proof that drinking wine or any other alcoholic beverage can replace these conventional measures.

The U.S. Food and Drug Administration warns that people who take aspirin regularly should not drink alcohol. Heart disease patients should stop drinking and continue aspirin if their doctor prescribed it for their heart condition. Patients should not stop taking aspirin without first talking to their doctor.

Cocaine

Cocaine abuse has been associated with a number of cardiovascular diseases such as cardiac arrhythmia, in which the normal rhythm of the heartbeat is disrupted. In severe cases of cardiac arrhythmia, death can occur, even in young people with no history of heart disease (NIDA 2005).

The National Institute on Drug Abuse (NIDA) Intramural Research Program (IRP) has discovered that certain compounds may be useful for treating cocaine-induced cardiac arrhythmia. The compounds block some of the actions of the chemical messenger serotonin in the heart (NIDA 1991).

Other researchers have shown that serotonin can elicit arrhythmia in human hearts. Since cocaine raises serotonin levels, among other actions, the IRP investigators reasoned that the serotonin-blocking compounds might be useful treatments for cardiac arrhythmia caused by cocaine abuse (Lucas and Ledgerwood 2004).

There are several effects of moderate cocaine use, such as disturbances in heart rhythm, increased heart and respiratory rates, elevated blood pressure, dilated pupils, decreased appetite, excessive activity, talkativeness, irritability, argumentative behavior, nervousness, or agitation. The effects of large amounts of cocaine cause a loss of coordination, collapse, perspiration, blurred vision, dizziness, feeling of restlessness, anxiety, delusions, heart attacks, chest pain, respiratory failure, strokes, seizures and headaches, abdominal pain, nausea, and paranoia (NIDA 1991, 2005).

Marijuana

Marijuana is the most widely used illegal substance in the world today (Johnston, O'Malley, and Bachman 2005). Its use is also the most controversial. With legalization efforts underway, it is important to have the facts of marijuana usage.

The majority of marijuana is smoked, although some users ingest it orally (added to brownies, cookies, etc.). Marijuana is usually smoked in the form of loosely rolled cigarettes called "joints," hollowed out commercial cigars called "blunts," or smoked in pipes or bongs. Joints and blunts are sometimes laced with a number of adulterants including PCP, cocaine, and embalming fluid (a chemical traditionally used to preserve dead bodies)—resulting in a wide range of effects.

Within a few minutes after inhaling marijuana smoke, an individual's heart begins to beat more rapidly, the bronchial passages relax and become enlarged, and blood vessels in the eyes expand, making the eyes look red. The heart rate, normally 70 to 80 beats per minute, may increase by 20 to 50 beats per minute or, in some cases, even double. This effect can be greater if other drugs are taken with marijuana (Mittleman et al. 2001).

The short-term effects of marijuana use include impairing short-term memory, concentration, attention, judgment, coordination, and balance. Marijuana also increases heart rate and causes blood shot or red eyes, dry mouth, and increased appetite (Brook, Rosen, and Brook 2001). The long-term effects of marijuana use include addiction (psychological), paranoia, persistent anxiety, impaired learning skills, and memory difficulties. Occasional effects, especially with long-term use, include anxiety, panic, and paranoia (Brook, Rosen, and Brook 2001).

There are a number of effects associated with marijuana use, including an increased risk of chronic cough, bronchitis, and emphysema; increased risk of cancer of the head, neck, and lungs; and a decrease in testosterone levels and lower sperm counts for men and an increase in testosterone levels for women and increased risk of infertility.

Finally, the ongoing use of marijuana has a devastating affect on cardiac transplant patients because the active chemical (THC) has a negative effect on the antirejection medications needed for transplant recovery. The use of marijuana after cardiac transplantation increases the chances of one's body rejecting the organ (SAMHA 2004).

PURPOSE/GOALS

The general purpose of a cardiac substance abuse group is three-fold. First, the purpose is to help the cardiac patient self-assess his or her level and severity of substance abuse. Second, it is to enhance the motivation and commitment to not self-medicate with licit and/or illicit substance. Finally, it is to help the cardiac patient develop an individualized plan of recovery. There is no singular plan of recovery. That is to say, the cardiac patient having a substance use disorder should develop a plan that minimizes the negative effects of licit and/or illicit substance abuse on furthering the patient's cardiac problems. Therefore, the options may include moderation management or sobriety, depending on the level of substance use severity.

FUNCTIONAL CHARACTERISTICS

The overall function of a cardiac substance use group is to help the cardiac patient self-assess his or her level or severity of substance use relative to its effect on current cardiac problems. This allows the cardiac patient to determine whether or not his or her current use will negatively effect, or exacerbate, the cardiac disease.

In this way, the cardiac substance abuse group is designed as educational and process-oriented. It is educational in the sense of providing cardiac patients cogent information so that they can make an informed decision as to how they wish to manage their use/abuse. Also, the cardiac substance group is a process entity in that it allows the individual cardiac patient to interact with others grappling with similar issues in assessing the relative effect of licit or illicit substance abuse on current cardiovascular disease.

Cardiac substance abuse groups are advantageous in several ways (Fisher 2004):

- Reduction in sense of isolation because there are other cardiac patients having similar problems
- Provision of positive peer support and pressures to either abstain from substances of abuse or modify their current use
- Enabling of cardiac patients who abuse substances to witness the recovery of others

- Provision of useful information to cardiac patients having substance abuse disorders
- Provision of directive feedback and negative critique needed to formulate a plan of recovery
- Offering of encouragement, support, and reinforcement that will reinforce cardiac patients' task of dealing with life "on life's terms"
- Provision of opportunities for the cardiac patient to develop and learn the social skills they need to cope with life
- Instillation of hope that change is possible
- Learning of alternative ways to cope with life stressors other than substance use/abuse
- Creation of a family-like experience to form a corrective emotional experience

STRUCTURAL CHARACTERISTICS

It is suggested that this group be structured as open-ended and heterogeneous relative to sex and cardiac disease. The rationale here is to allow cardiac patients to interact in a way that allows individuals to confront one another's severity of substance use relative to managing their cardiac problems. Within this framework, cardiac patients having substance abuse disorders can assess their situation on an individual basis, against other members and relative to their outcome expectations.

The model suggested for treatment of cardiac substance use disorder is one that is synthesized: cognitive-behavioral (Fisher 1995, 2004) and motivation interviewing (Miller and Rollnick 1991). The rationale is that most individuals diagnosed with cardiac disease have only a minimal understanding of the severity of their substance use and have lesser understanding of the net impact of the substance used as a contributory factor in cardiac disease.

Motivational interviewing techniques help the cardiac patient self-assess, using a cost-benefit analysis of the severity of his or her substance use, and help to promote healthy changes (i.e., either abstinence or modification of substances used). The cognitive-behavioral method helps the client confront the reality of substance use/abuse on the overall outcome of one's cardiac disease. In addition, the use of cognitive-behavioral techniques helps the cardiac patient develop a "safety plan" (i.e., alternative ways to minimize the net impact of substances on worsening the cardiac disease process).

GROUP LEADERSHIP SKILLS

The social group worker has to have specialized training in both the principles of cognitive-behavioral techniques and motivational interviewing, as well as a comprehensive understanding of the motivational stages of change. The social group worker leading a cardiac substance abuse group needs to be comfortable with resistance, overt defensiveness, and ambivalence. In addition, he or she needs to have a healthy respect for the cardiac patient's sense of self-determination, even when this is diametrically different from what the cardiac professionals believe to be a healthy course for the patient.

The social group worker needs to have a complete understanding of the stages of change, so that an accurate assessment can be made of the motivational level of each client referred for substance abuse treatment. As cardiac patients move through different stages of recovery, the treatment approach should move with them. That is to say, the therapeutic strategies and level of direct participation by the social group work will change with the conditions of the patients.

In the beginning phase of treatment, patients, especially cardiac patients, tend to be ambivalent about ending substance use. Furthermore, the patients tend to be rigid in their thought processing, and fairly limited in their ability to solve problems. The art of intervening with cardiac patients in this early stage is centered on the healthy confrontation of denial and resistance. During this phase, the cardiac patient having a substance use disorder is typically more receptive to peers than professionals have. That is, information from peers in a social group is more easily accepted than from a lone clinical professional.

Cardiac patients in the middle phase of substance abuse treatment remain vulnerable. During this phase of treatment, the cardiac patient having substance abuse problems may recall the comfort and familiarity of their substance abuse, but forget just how bad the rest of their lives were. This is where the social group worker acts as an anchor relative to the reality of the patients' substance use experiences. During this phase, the cardiac patient having a substance use disorder is at a greater risk for a lapse (return to the substance, but with a realization that this is not a healthy or helpful place to stay) or relapse (the cardiac substance abuser returns to his or her premorbid level and severity of use). Since cardiac patients with substance abuse typically are isolated from healthy social groups, the cardiac substance abuse group helps acculturate cardiac patients into a culture of recovery. The social group worker draws attention to positive developments, notes how the cardiac patient has progressed, and affirms the possibility of enhanced and increased connection as a positive outcome.

In the ending phase of substance abuse treatment, cardiac patients are stable enough to confront situations that involve conflict or deep emotion. At this point of treatment, a process-oriented social group may become appropriate for some patients who finally are able to confront emotionally painful realities (e.g., history of being a child or adult child of an alcoholic or drug addict, history of abuse, etc.). Other cardiac patients may need the substance group to help them develop healthier interpersonal relationships with significant others, enhance communication in a more direct fashion, or develop more appropriate roles such as spouse or parent.

CLINICAL TECHNIQUES UTILIZED

The social group worker needs to have an advanced understanding of cognitive-behavioral techniques especially related to the development of alternative and healthier coping skills. In addition, the social group worker needs a comprehensive working knowledge of motivational interviewing and the stages of change.

The stages of change model shows that, for most persons, a change in behavior occurs gradually, with the patient moving from being uninterested, unaware, or unwilling to make a change (precontemplation), to considering a change (contemplation), to deciding and preparing to make a change. Genuine, determined action is then taken and, over time, attempts to maintain the new behavior occur. Relapses are almost inevitable and become part of the process of working toward lifelong change. See Chapter 4 for an overview of the five stages of change: precontemplation, contemplation, preparative, action and maintenance, and relapse prevention.

The stages of change model encompasses many concepts from previously developed models (Prochaska and DiClemente 1992). The health belief model (Rosenstock 1974), the locus of control model (Lefcourt and Davidson-Katz 1991), and behavioral models (Skinner 1950) fit together well within this framework. During the precontemplation stage, patients do not consider change. They may not believe that their behavior is a problem or that it will negatively affect them (health belief model), or they may be resigned to their unhealthy behavior because of previous failed efforts and no longer believe that they have control (external locus of control). During the contemplation stage, patients struggle with ambivalence, weighing the pros and cons of their current behavior and the benefits of and barriers to change (health belief model). Cognitive-behavioral models of change (e.g., focusing on coping skills or environmental manipulation) and twelve-step programs fit well in the preparation, action, and maintenance stages (Fisher 1995). Motivational interviewing techniques (Miller and Rollnick 1991) help the cardiac patient self-assess what stage he or she is in relative to willingness to change (e.g., moderate alcohol and drug use, quitting all substance use). Socratic questioning and reflexive and responsive listening and interaction help the cardiac patient with substance abuse or dependency problem self-assess his or her outcome expectations in relation to his or her health and cardiac recovery.

In addition, the social group worker needs advance skills in helping the cardiac substance abuse patient to develop an individualized plan of recovery. The social group worker needs to help the cardiac patient identify feelings, both positive and negative, and areas of major stress; detect the underlying negative thoughts, ideations, and perceptions that contribute to negative feelings and stressors; and actively challenge and reframe negative thoughts, ideations, and structuring negative perceptions for which the patient is self-medicating. In addition, the clinical social needs to help the cardiac patient develop prosocial problems-solving methods and interpersonal decision making skills by using a cost-benefit self-assessment of outcome expectations. The social group worker needs to help the patient develop an individualized plan of recovery. There is no one outcome for the patient concerning substance use and abuse. The cardiac patient may wish, based on assessment, to modify substance use or enter into sobriety.

The social group worker needs to have a thorough understanding of the two major models of substance abuse treatment: the disease-and-recovery model and the cognitive-behavioral model. From the perspective of the disease-and-recovery model, the only worthwhile outcome is complete sobriety, which is attained from using a twelve-step approach. The disease-and-recovery model conceptualizes the substance use disorder as a disease over which the cardiac patient is powerless (Fisher 1995, 2004). In the cognitive-behavior model, the substance use disorder is conceptualized as a problem of self-medication for painful emotional and/or physical pain. The cognitive-behavioral model is an empowerment approach, which supports that the cardiac patient is in control, at least over the first use. Hence, the cardiac patient can choose modification of substance use or sobriety (Fisher 1995, 2004). (For an analysis of the effectiveness of the disease-and-recovery model and the cognitive-behavioral model in both an inpatient and outpatient setting, the reader is referred to Fisher and Bentley's 1996 research.)

EXPECTED CLINICAL BENEFITS AND OUTCOMES

The expected and anticipated outcomes are:

1. Enhancement of the cardiac patient's understanding of substance use in general relative to its impact on specific cardiac diseases
2. Enhancement of the cardiac patient's motivation to deal practically with his or her substance use and make the critical connection between substance abuse and current cardiac disease and/or worsening of the cardiac disease
3. Development of a plan to manage the cardiac patient's substance use either through moderation management or sobriety
4. Development of an individualized recovery plan, based on the individual cardiac patient's motivation and willingness to change
5. Assessment of the overall impact of substance use on the quality and duration of one's life as a cardiac patient
6. Gaining an understanding of the how the use of substances influences the patient's significant others

CONCLUSIONS

The involvement of cardiac patients evaluated as having a substance use disorder, either abuse (a judgment problem) or dependency (a psychosocial and/or physical addiction), in a social group context helps the patient self-assess his or her understanding of licit or illicit substance use/abuse relative to the management of their cardiac recovery. In addition, through the use of both cognitive-behavioral and motivational interviewing techniques, the cardiac patient is able to make informed decisions about the role of substance abuse in his or her life. Often, providing cogent and reliable information about the effects of various substances on the body helps to improve one's willingness to alter his or her lifestyle.

Chapter 13

Human Sexuality for Cardiac Patients

INTRODUCTION

Humans are sexual beings throughout their life span. Early in each person's development and psychosocial socialization, an individual begins to view himself or herself as a sexual being, complete with culturally linked gender role expectations. It is clear to all humans that sex and reproduction have a clear and unmistakable link. Human sexuality is poorly understood and therefore rarely explained in general and specifically is not dealt with when one is dealing with a major medical disease.

Yet, to be sure, beyond one's income, political, and religious preferences, sexuality is the most personal, private, and sensitive aspect of an individual's being. Socially, how one defines his or her sexuality is quite individualized. It has been stated that one's sexuality is "as individualized as one's fingerprint; there are no two heterosexuals or homosexuals who have the same sexual preferences" (Pranzarone 1978). To say the least, one's sexuality is a complex and extremely personal area of his or her life.

Generally, individuals prefer to define human sexuality as the thoughts, feelings, responses, and reactions that one's body and "brain" have to situations and events, which may or may not lead to the completion of "the sex act." Human libido has been described in many different ways, but appears often to be confused with lust and desire and is often thought to have various levels of excitement or response. Sex is something that men and women both think about or at least it comes to mind with a great degree of frequency, depending on an unending series of occasions, times, and places.

Social Group Work with Cardiac Patients
© 2007 by The Haworth Press, Inc. All rights reserved.
doi:10.1300/5739_13

RATIONALE FOR USING
THE SOCIAL GROUP WORK MODEL

In an attempt to demystify much that surrounds human sexuality and healthy cardiovascular function, the American Health Association has elected to maintain an awareness campaign on cardiovascular health and disease. It is based on a recent academic and research outcome (e.g., Papadopoulous 1989), which described human sexuality as having incredible benefits for cardiac health, stress relief, prevention of cancers, increased longevity, along with other physical and emotional benefits. The Society for the Scientific Study of Sexuality released their "white paper" on the subject (West, Vinikoor, and Zolnoun 2004).

It is interesting that the same organ is the center of both so much anxiety about death and the center of our passion for life—symbolically known as the heart. The math is simple: many individuals talk to their doctor about cardiac risk, but few people talk to their doctor about sex. Almost no one talks to their doctor about both.

The area of cardiac health and sexuality is an uncertain one. There are facts, opinions, and a distinct lack of reliable information that would be helpful to both patients and physicians. At least one million Americans have a heart attack each year. It appears that these are almost never precipitated by sexual activity (Sipski and Alexander 1997). However, no one is really certain what "almost never" means. There have been no controlled studies yielding reliable data. For starters, people do not always tell the truth when reporting about sexual activities. More to the point, professional institutions are particularly uninterested in commissioning studies about the sexual aspects of health care. As a result, physicians and patients have to make educated guesses about this central aspect of physical and mental health.

It is also hard to measure the impact of sexual activity on cardiac function because the content and impact of sexual activity varies greatly from person to person over time. For some people, thirty minutes of sex involves ten seconds of rather sedentary intercourse, while for others, it involves twenty-nine minutes of vigorous thrusting and other energetic activities (Papadopoulous 1989; Schwartz and Rodriguez 2005).

Some individuals believe that extramarital or other illicit sexual activities such as going to prostitutes increase the risk of cardiac events. One of the few studies to actually look at this is a recent Japanese study albeit with a flawed methodology. It may be counterintuitive, but a prostitute in a hotel with a naked dead guy is probably more likely to report sexual activity ("it wasn't murder, it was sex") than a wife, who would presumably be quite distraught and want a civil face for investigators. Thus, biased reporting can exaggerate the cardiac dangers of illicit sex.

Orgasm itself would appear to carry virtually no risk for a heart attack. It typically occurs gradually enough so that severe pain would stop it before it became too dangerous. Orgasm itself probably poses more vascular than cardiac danger, since one often holds one's breath and raises intracranial pressure (Schwartz and Rodriguez 2005).

Finally, risk factors need to be understood in practical context. In truth, food, alcohol, cigarettes, and emotional stress pose far more dangers than sex (Schwartz and Rodriguez 2005). So does crossing the street, statistically speaking, especially when an individual is distracted by lighting a cigarette or buttering toast.

The treatment for cardiac care poses an entirely different set of sexual challenges. The most common medications—beta-blockers, calcium channel blockers, diuretics, and ACE inhibitors—often contribute to erection problems. Underline "contribute," because many men are frightened enough after a heart attack to create erection problems independent of medication. Similarly, the partner (male or female) of someone who has had a heart attack may be frightened enough that she or he may unintentionally help create the circumstances for erection problem through expressed concern or fear for the patient, anxiety, criticism, rigidity, or withdrawal. If drugs are suspected in postheart attack sexual difficulties, a physician should experiment with the dosage, timing, or type of drug. If the erection or ejaculation problem looks as if it has a psychological component, a patient should be referred to a mental health professional or sex therapist. To help patients follow the referral, describe it as an important, standard part of cardiac care follow-up. And, the health care professional should inquire about patients concerning any other drugs they are taking, either licit or illicit, prescribed or not (Schwartz and Rodriguez 2005). For example, the real culprit might be, say, an antidepressant or mood stabilizing medication that the patient forgot to mention.

Obviously, social workers and other professionals involved in cardiac treatment should tell patients to monitor their bodies for signs of trouble. Pain always means stop, or at least slow down. But many warning signs of cardiac problems—shortness of breath, rapid pulse, disorientation, sweating, chest pressure—commonly accompany sexual arousal. Professionals don't want to alarm patients needlessly, nor have them constricting their sexual expression unnecessarily.

Finally, a few words about medications prescribed to enhance sexual performance such as Viagra. Various patients find this to be a marriage-saver, a disappointment, or the source of problems. Viagra is contraindicated in patients using nitrates—and that's at least five million men. It is important to emphasize this for patients, even if they're not taking Viagra at the moment. If they are, remind them, and have them tell their partners (assuming that their partners know that they are taking Viagra, which again is another story). Therefore, in essence, since human sexuality is a psychosocial as well as a biologic imperative, it falls within the clinical domain of social group work.

PURPOSE/GOALS

Human sexuality is a psychological, social, and biological aspect of life. The purpose of intervening in this aspect of the cardiac patient's life is predicated upon the lifelong role that sexuality plays in an individuals' daily life. After a heart attack or other cardiac event, an early goal is to climb a flight of stairs in thirty to sixty seconds. A cardiac patient will begin an exercise program after tests show the heart is healing. Cardiac patients are warned not to exercise after eating to avoid fatigue.

Because of such caution toward physical activity after a heart attack, many couples mistakenly believe intercourse is risky and abstain from it. Couples may also avoid holding, caressing, or pleasuring because they think these activities may lead to intercourse. Unfortunately, these fears may place a strain on their lives and their relationships.

Heart attacks and other cardiac diseases differ widely in severity. Many men and women recover with little damage. Today, individuals with heart attacks, or other cardiovascular illnesses once considered damaging, can be treated with surgery and medications and then return to reasonably normal lives. Most people who have had heart attacks and other cardiac maladies can return to their careers.

In addition to work, sexuality is important to an individual's self-esteem. Men and women who are not informed about the potential for living nearly normal lives, including enjoying a normal sexual life, may become fearful and depressed and adopt a lifelong defeatist outlook. It is important to receive sexual instructions before and after discharge from the hospital, or cardiac rehabilitation programs, to counter unwarranted fears that might hinder the cardiac patient from enjoying a full life.

Total rehabilitation after a heart attack includes sexual rehabilitation, an aspect of recovery that should not be overlooked. And, since sexual relationships are, by their nature, social interactions, it becomes fodder for social group workers.

FUNCTIONAL CHARACTERISTICS

Since sexual interaction and involvement is a social construct as much as it is a biological imperative, social work groups serve a dualistic role. That is to educate cardiac patients and their significant other about sexuality as it relates to cardiovascular disease, and to process the impact and difficulties that cardiac patients and their significant others are experiencing. Relative to the educational aspect, the social group worker needs to address the limits of sexual activity related to cardiovascular illness, and the sundry prescribed medications that can cause compromised sexuality activity.

Relative to the process aspects, the social group worker will need to help cardiac patients and their significant others address general and specific concerns about sexuality postcardiac event, as well as specifically how the individual cardiac patient experiences sexuality.

STRUCTURAL CHARACTERISTICS

The social group on cardiac sexuality can be either homogeneous or heterogeneous relative to the sex mix in the group. Typically, these groups utilize a heterogeneous mix of cardiac patients and their significant others or partners. This allows patients and their loved ones to develop their specific concerns.

In general, it is suggested that these groups meet on at least a weekly basis. This type of social group begins with an agenda or topic and allows time for the patients and their significant others to have time during the latter part of the group to grapple with how to utilize presented information and to raise specific areas of concern.

There are at least five topical areas of education that needs to be addressed.

General Outcome Effects of Cardiovascular Disease on Sexual Activity

- Specific cardiac diseases' effect on sexuality
- General issues and differences between how men and women experience sexuality

Relationship of Cardiac Medications on Sexual Behavior and Outcome

- Beta-blockers
- Calcium blocker
- Blood thinners
- Blood pressure medications

Relationship of Other Medications on Sexual Behavior and Outcome

Medications can interfere with sexual function and satisfaction in a number of ways. The following list, although not exhaustive, includes commonly prescribed drugs that have been implicated as affecting sexual functioning:

(*Note:* Tranquilizers, such as Valium and Librium, and alcohol may increase sexual desire among inhibited individuals, but diminish both arousal and orgasm.)

Antihypertensive Drugs (Drugs Used to Treat High Blood Pressure)

- Thiazide diuretics-blockers (Propranol, Atenolol, Pindolol)
- Clonidine

- Guanethidine
- Alpha methyldopa
- Prozasin
- Hydralazine
- Reserpine
- Spironolactone

Psychoactive Agents (Drugs Used to Treat Depression, Anxiety, Insomnia, and Other Psychological Conditions)

- Tricyclic antidepressants
- Imipramine
- Doxepin
- Amitryptyline
- Major tranquilizers (Chlorpromazine, Butyrophenone, Prochlorperazine, Perpheasine, Trifluoperazine, Thioridazine)
- Monoamine oxidase inhibitors (Pargyline, Phenelzine)

Other Drugs

- Digoxin
- Cimetidine
- Clofibrate
- Blofibrate

Drugs Used in Cancer Chemotherapy

- Acetazolamide
- Heparin
- Estrogen
- Anorectic agents

Psychosocial Aspects of Having Cardiac Disease on Sexual Activities

- Patient-focused discussion of anxiety, concerns, and fears about engaging in sexual activity after a cardiac event
- Significant others' discussion of anxiety, concerns, and fears about engaging in sexual activities after a cardiac event
- Realistic versus unrealistic expectancies

Understanding of Psychosexual Medications on Cardiac Patients

There are now three oral erectile dysfunction (ED) drugs; Viagra, (sildenafil) by Pfizer; Levitra (vardenafil) by Bayer Pharmaceutical and Glaxo-Smith-Kline-Beecham/Schering Plough; and Cialis (tadalafil) by LillyICOS.

The dilemma is which drug to choose and why. For all practical purposes, these drugs—including Viagra, Levitra, and Cialis—are the first line of oral treatment for males with erectile dysfunction, in certain circumstances, in which the males are young with no comorbidities. (Here, comorbidities are defined as conditions that exist at the same time as the primary condition in the same patient [i.e., hypertension is a comorbidity of many conditions such as diabetes, ischemic heart disease, and end-stage renal disease]). Once a CVD is diagnosed and stabilized (e.g., laboratory tests are considered normal), one should look for the etiology of his erectile dysfunction before instituting treatment, since the disease process may be more serious than the symptoms, that is, the ED itself. In some cases, treatment of the primary disease may in fact resolve the sexual dysfunction. However, most men have a cause for their ED as noted by the history, the physical examination, the laboratory tests, and PDE-5 inhibitors are the first line of choice.

Selection of the preferred medication for treatment of sexual dysfunction should include a thorough history of the presenting patient and his partner. Description of the most frequently used medications, along with rationale for selection of the drug of choice in treatment situations, is presented as follows.

Viagra

Viagra was the first and is probably the most famous of the three PDE-5 inhibitors used to treat erectile dysfunction. Initially, there was concern about cardiovascular deaths; however, with time it is obvious that this drug is extremely safe when used correctly. Of the three drugs discussed here, Viagra has been on the market the longest, with the most medications and the most sexual situations of any of the three. It works in about 70 percent of all men with all types of erectile dysfunction, although approximately 25 percent of them do not feel that the responses are optimal. Its major drawbacks have been decreased absorption due to food intake, and, therefore, it is advised to take the Viagra on an empty stomach having no food for two to three hours prior to taking the pill and waiting at least one hour for sexual stimulation, but no longer than four hours, and obviously sexual stimulation is necessary. Absorption of Viagra is affected by food; it takes approximately thirty minutes to begin absorption, one hour to reach maximal concentration, and loses 50 percent of its highest concentration every four hours. Of the three drugs, the maximal concentration for Viagra appears to be the therapeutic concentration, which is not true of the other two drugs (Lewis, Rosen, and Goldstein 2005; Whitehill 2005; Kloner 2004).

Levitra

Levitra was the second oral PDE-5 inhibitor for erectile dysfunction to be approved by the Food and Drug Administration (FDA). Studies done on Levitra have excluded patients who failed Viagra, and therefore the efficacies are somewhat shifted toward the positive. In general, the feeling is that Levitra is more potent and efficient than Viagra, as demonstrated by the hard-to-treat groups of patients. Diabetics and post-radical-nerve-sparing-prostatectomy patients appear to have a higher incidence of efficacy than for Viagra. In addition, the efficacy is based on sexual satisfaction or successful penetration rather than improvement, which were the endpoints for Viagra. Levitra reaches its peaks concentration at forty minutes, and is affected only by a very high fat diet, and therefore, most patients can eat with the drug without affecting its absorption and maximal concentration (Lewis et al. 2005; Whitehill 2005; Kloner 2004).

The half-life of Levitra is five hours; however, the therapeutic levels appear not to be the maximal concentration. Therefore, multiple half-lives may occur with efficacy of the drug. Overall, the slight chemical change noted in Levitra appears to give it more potency, efficacy, longer duration, and probably more rapid onset. Levitra has shown that 25 percent of their patients had optimal responses within sixteen minutes of the oral intake of the pill. When talking about duration, however, Cialis appears to be the winner (Lewis et al. 2005; Kloner 2004).

Cialis

Cialis has been approved for duration of thirty-six hours; however, there are studies showing high efficacy out to 100 hours. It is not affected by any food whatsoever and in fact can be taken with pure fat. Viagra, on the other hand, is impeded by any type of food and Levitra absorption is impeded by a high-fat diet in which more than 62 percent of the fat and the calories are from fat. The typical double cheeseburger with french fries and malted milkshake would certainly inhibit the effect of Levitra, but a steak with potatoes, a glass of wine, salad, and dessert would probably not. Neither of these would affect the absorption of Cialis. Cialis is protein-bound and, therefore, has a serum peak concentration at two hours and a half-life anywhere between sixteen and twenty-two hours, depending on the age of the patient. The older the patient, the longer the half-life. The long duration of action, the lack of absorption effects, and efficacy at least as good as Viagra, if not better than, and probably almost as good as Levitra, make Cialis a unique and different drug. Cialis is the true "weekend" erectile dysfunction drug (Lewis et al. 2005; Whitehill 2005; Kloner 2004).

GROUP LEADERSHIP SKILLS

Beyond the fundamental aspects of understanding and utilizing social group work methods, the clinical social worker needs to have a replete and comprehensive understanding of human sexuality, including sexuality related to chronic medical conditions, especially cardiovascular; an appreciation and recognition of how various ethno-cultures and different racial groups manage sexuality; and an appreciation of the differences about how males versus female deal with sexuality and sexual dysfunction.

Equally important is that the social group worker needs to be comfortable dealing with and managing sexuality. Thus, the professional social group worker needs to be fairly comfortable in discussing and dealing with sexual topics. This requires the social group worker to be in touch and comfortable with his or her own sexual identity and have a comfort level with the topical material.

Since many individuals in medical and/or psychosocial treatment have a poor socialized sex model due to inadequate parenting and family-of-origin dysfunction, it is advisable to have coleadership in this social group. That is to say, ideally, this social group would have a male and female coleadership construction, so as model-appropriate, healthy sex roles, and also to help patients of either sex gain some level of psychosexual comfort and ability to address relevant issues, the workers can raise appropriate questions and be positioned to better understand the material presented through dealing with social group members of the opposite sex. (That is, this facilitates patients of both sexes to develop a level of comfort and be able to understand sexual issues from different points of worldview.) Finally, given the intense and personal nature of the topical area of this type of group, it is quite helpful to be involved in direct supervision so as to maintain one's objective stance, and also to deal with the social group worker's potential transference (feeling and thoughts that the patient projects onto the social worker) and countertransference (feelings and thoughts that the social worker projects onto the patient) issues as they evolve and mature in the group. These issues need to be monitored through supervision because of the intense and intimate nature of the topic and the potentiality that either the social worker and/or the cardiac patient may identify or develop emotional attachments that can prove unhealthy.

CLINICAL TECHNIQUES UTILIZED

The social group worker will need to have specialized skills in understanding the fundamentals of human sexuality, and also an ongoing supervision as to how the social group worker is self-managing his or her own sexuality. In addition, the social group worker will need to develop a replete understanding of his or her own views of responsible sexual behaviors, and also develop a comfort zone about his or her sexuality. That is to say, the social group worker needs to have a healthy handle on his or her own sexuality and be able to tolerate and be sensitive to alternative sexual behaviors without being punitive, moralistic, or judgmental.

Professional social group workers need to develop not only awareness, but also a true sensitivity toward issues related to sexuality in service delivery by:

- *Holding professional clinical staff meetings and supervision.* Everyone within the cardiac rehabilitation program—from aides to professionals, to medical staff, to administrators—is part of the team. All staff within the cardiac rehabilitation program benefit from periodic orientation to basic clinic services and critical topics such as sexuality and sexual health.
- *Raising staff awareness.* Identify colleagues working in the area of gender and sexuality, and invite them to meet with your staff to help raise staff awareness of gender and sexuality. Use this as a first step for enhancing the client responsiveness of service the social group worker delivers, with support from supervision.
- *Being a good role model.* The social group worker is in a powerful position to set a good example. Model good behavior during the course of the day, and encourage all cardiac rehabilitation staff and colleagues to do the same.

EXPECTED CLINICAL BENEFITS AND OUTCOMES

The general expected outcome of cardiac patients and significant behaviors involved in a social group devoted to addressing sexuality after a cardiac event include, but are not limited to, the following:

1. Development of healthy postcardiac event sexual expectations
2. The limits of sexual behavior relative to specific cardiovascular illnesses
3. Signs and symptoms of sexual behavior that may trigger medical attention
4. An understanding of the various medications and medical procedures that negatively affect the cardiac patient's sexuality
5. An understanding of the current "state-of-the-art" medications that can improve sexual performance
6. Appreciation of the limitations of one's sexuality after a cardiac event

7. An ability to discern sensuality versus sexuality
8. An understanding of the psychosocial and medical limitation with which one has to contend relative to specific cardiovascular illnesses
9. Breaking down and developing an understanding of myths, folkways, and urban legends versus pragmatic sexual limitations of cardiovascular illness

CONCLUSIONS

A person's sexuality is as unique as one's fingerprint. No two individuals who profess and practice the same general sexual interest have the same specific needs (i.e., what he or she finds enjoyable, sensual, and sexually satisfying). In the best of times, and under relatively normal conditions, one's sexuality and the discussion of it, is extremely sensitive and personal. Often, individuals are either ashamed or embarrassed to deal with this topic depending on how they were socialized in their family-of-origin. This is particularly true when one is struggling with a major cardiovascular disease. Through involvement in a social group, one can learn usable information and process how this can be used in their interpersonal sexual lives. Much fear and angst can be allayed by one's involvement in this social group. In addition, the group members will develop a natural support with fellow members, and be able to share and normalize experiences.

Chapter 14

Cardiac Support Groups

INTRODUCTION

A chronic health condition or prolonged illness, such as cardiovascular disease, affects many aspects of a person's life. The support of friends, family, and health care providers is important as the cardiac patient learn to cope with these changes. The advice and support of those who have had similar experiences can also be beneficial. Most cardiac rehabilitation programs typically offer a number of targeted support groups for patients with cardiovascular disease. In these forums, participants will have opportunities to learn more about their conditions, share their experiences, and address their questions and concerns.

Traditionally, support groups have been utilized in a variety of health care settings and with myriad individuals in mental health, substance abuse treatment, and in health care settings. Within the context of health care settings, support groups have been effectively utilized with cancer patients, individuals with potentially life-threatening diseases, and with patients diagnosed with cardiovascular disease. Some of these support groups are self-supporting by the members and others have the involvement of a professional to help with operational issues and development of cogent content. The typical goals of these support groups include focus on the following: emotional support, resource information, educational, and self-advocacy (Betz et al. 1990; Myers 1995; Rollins 1987).

Social Group Work with Cardiac Patients
© 2007 by The Haworth Press, Inc. All rights reserved.
doi:10.1300/5739_14

DIFFERENCES BETWEEN SUPPORT GROUPS
AND SOCIAL GROUP WORK MODELS

As delineated in a previous work (Fisher 2004), it is imperative to differentiate between social groups and self-help, support groups. Social group work is defined as:

> An orientation and methods of social work in intervention in which small numbers of people who share similar interests or concerns [e.g., relative to an identity such as cardiac patient] or problems, convene regularly and engage in activities designed to achieve their common goals. In contrast to group psychother-apy, the goals of group work are not necessarily the treatment of emotional problems. Their objectives also include exchanging information, developing social and manual skills, changing value orientation, and diverting [maladaptive] behaviors into productive channels. Interventive techniques include, but are not limited to, controlled therapeutic discussions . . . education, and tutoring. (Baker 1999, p. 449)

Social group work models in health care stress the difficulties that members have in integrating and modulating their affective lives. In contrast to self-help, support groups are conducted by practitioners who use a psychosocial model of treatment on which to base deci-sions about group composition, interventive strategies, and therapeutic goals. Other group experiences, such as self-help, supportive groups, may provide crucial support members who experience period of pain-ful uncovering in-group work. Hence, it is possible to see other groups complimenting the efforts of group work (Fisher 1994). Yet, it is im-portant to note that support groups are not treatment per se; they are ancillary and collateral to treatment efforts and prove helpful for a person who lacks a supportive interpersonal network.

Self-help groups are a growing phenomenon across national borders and sociopolitical systems. These groups affect individual participants' activity levels in medical programs such as cardiac rehabilitation, and also serve to strengthen their self-perception along with a sense of be-longing. In this vein, support groups have played a vital role in health care in general and specifically in cardiac psychosocial rehabilita-tion. Katz and Bender (1976) were among the first to question the connection between self-help groups and professional involvement. This author noted that as therapeutic and physical extenders of services, self-help groups are significant adjuncts to more formal professionally led social groups.

In a sociological study conducted by Adamsen and Rasmussen (2001), they researched the impact of support group having professional staff involvement with those that were conducted by patients only. These researchers showed that health care professionals, such as social workers, nurses, and psychologist, have increasingly become an integral part of self-help groups in health settings. Involvement in self-help groups is a relatively new role for helping professionals. Hence, these researchers suggest a reassessment of the operational aspects of self-help groups with a focus on using health care professionals in a consultative role.

RATIONALE FOR USING THE SOCIAL GROUP WORK MODEL

There are numerous efficacious reasons for using a support group for cardiac patients. The least of which is the psychosocial need for an individual experiencing a potential life-threatening event so decrease isolation, increase identification, and enhance feelings of hope. Other incentives for the use of cardiac support groups include, but are not limited to the following:

- A cardiac support group can offer emotional support to those who have experienced a heart problem, and they offer an opportunity for members to share a common or difficult experience in their individual lives.
- A support group can maintain ongoing rehabilitation and secondary prevention, keeping members current with healthy lifestyle recommendations.
- A heart support group can direct people to services that are already established, and are of value to heart patients, such as stop smoking clinics, healthy eating demonstrations, and stress management courses.

Groups offer valuable support to partners, significant others, and family members. It has the same level of enthusiasm, and in the same way that heart patients receive support to express their fears and anxieties and learn how others have coped in similar situations. This helps reduce the patient's sense of isolation.

Heart support groups complement the services already offered by health care professionals. A heart support group does not set out to replace any existing services, but is another way to access a kind of help that is unavailable elsewhere.

A cardiac support group has an enhanced probability of being successful, as it is has been established in response to a clinically identified need. For this reason, many cardiac support groups have tended to be specialized depending on the type of cardiovascular illness and the support needs for that patient population. Therefore, prior to starting a cardiac support group, it is recommended that the social group worker use either formal or informal methods to determine need for a specific support group. In a formal approach, the social worker may contact patients and their respective family members via in-person interviews, telephone interviews, or by pursuing a questionnaire methodology. Once the cardiac patients and their family members have highlighted their supportive needs, then the social worker can synthesize this input. Less formal methods of establishing a support group need to meet with various stakeholders, including cardiologist, cardiac nurses, recreational therapist, nutritionists, as well as any other cardiac rehabilitation staff involved in direct cardiac treatment. In addition, the social group worker can gain valuable input about the need for specific cardiac support by conducting focus groups with the patients, former patients, their respective family members, and significant others involved in the patients' lives. Various specialized cardiac support groups may include: individuals who have experienced any type of cardiac condition; a general type of groups; individuals with specific cardiac problems, such as heart failure, or patients who have a particular device such as a pacemaker or an implantable cardioverter defibrillator (ICD); patients who have been diagnosed with a cardiac problem or who have already had an operation on their heart or circulatory system, and who are interested in maintaining a healthy heart and improved lifestyle; family members, significant others, and those who provide care within the family; and parents of children living with a heart condition.

PURPOSE/GOALS

Depending on the type of cardiovascular illness and the patients involved, the specific purpose and support group goals will vary. For example, if one is setting up a cardiac support group for patients who are postoperative, the purpose of the group may include normalizing the aftereffects of the surgical procedures, sharing feeling and thoughts about the potential barriers and obstacles to cardiac recovery, gain some pragmatic understanding from other cardiac patients about limitation placed on them by their disease process, and/or the affects the heart problem has had on their families. Family members and significant others may utilize a support group to discuss the effects of the identified cardiac patient's condition on the family-as-a-whole, sharing resource information, and helping one another understand their unique role in the rehabilitation process.

Irrespective of the specifics of conducting a cardiac support group, there are some core goals inherent in all such groups. Surveys of families and health care professionals dealing with major diseases have identified the following general goals (Adamsen and Rasmussen 2001; Adamsen 2002; Shulman 1983). These goals, clustered in three different domains, can be used when starting a support group but must be adapted and expanded according to the group's specific needs.

Emotional Support Goals

- Provide encouragement, hope, and help to the cardiac patients and families in need.
- Decrease feelings of isolation.
- Reduce anxiety and stress for the cardiac patients and their family members.
- Increase coping skills.

Resource Information Goals

- Gather and share information.
- Identify and increase available resources for cardiac patients and their individual families.

Educational Goals

Provide information on congenital and/or acquired heart disease, diagnostic procedures, medications, cardiac coping behaviors necessary for recovery, and hospitalization issues, through professional health care resources.

Cardiac support groups must identify the strategies for each goal and the persons responsible for carrying them out. The four support group methods for meeting these goals are educational, mutual-peer support, educational-mutual support, and ventilation.

FUNCTIONAL CHARACTERISTICS

Obviously, the core function of a cardiac support group is to develop methods for self-help with guidance from a professional social group worker. Although it is suggested that a professional group worker be involved in the planning, design, development, and operational aspects of cardiac support groups, the group members themselves have to identify individuals from within the group to carry out specific tasks, and accept various roles (i.e., seeking informal and formal resources). The core operation of the cardiac support group is built on mutual aid among the memberships.

STRUCTURAL CHARACTERISTICS

Cardiac support groups can be either informal or formal. In an informal group, all members tend to make decisions together, rather than relying a committee or professional. There is usually no one person in the role of chair, secretary, or treasurer. In the informal support group, it is important that tasks and roles be shared around the group, and that no one individual gets "stuck" with all the responsibility. Pooling resources and working together will make the cardiac support group psychosocially stronger and vital. Often, within an informal support group the leadership for each session is rotated.

As informal cardiac support groups grow and develop over time, some opt to become more formalized. Often the rationale for this move is to legitimize the support group within either the outpatient or hospital-based organization. Also, the formalization of support groups moves them to a different level of funding, that is to say, if the support group is in need of money or other concrete resources, such as educational material or fund to pay for professional speakers, informal groups may move to link itself to an organization.

For cardiac support groups to be formalized, the structure will have to change. The peer leadership has to be designated by formal vote or appointment by the group-as-a-whole. In addition, oftentimes, the group will move to have written protocols (i.e., meeting agendas, by-laws, role definitions, and policy, and procedures to guide its direction). Two advantages for these written protocols are that it gives the group a sense of professionalism and allows the group to legitimatize itself for both host organization and outside source funding.

Creating a Cardiac Support Group

Establish a Projected Time Line

The following tasks must be completed for successful implementation of a cardiac support group:

- Determine the goals and focus of the group (write a twenty-to thirty-word statement of purpose and philosophy is suggested for clarity and conciseness).
- Name the group (*note:* this is important to making the support group both appealing as well as acceptable to the community at large).
- Elect officers or fill positions.
- Set up committees.
- Write bylaws (optional).
- Apply for tax-exempt (nonprofit) status (optional).
- Cover legal checkpoints (liability and tax issues) (optional).

Determine Program Priorities

This will serve to guide the group in terms of membership, advocacy activities, and respectability within the community.

GROUP LEADERSHIP SKILLS

The role of the social group worker in a cardiac support group is basically defined by the group's purpose. Generally, the professional's role will be to give guidance, direction, and support relative to gathering resources and resource development. Typically, there are two types of leadership styles that the social group work can provide:

1. *Passive-participant leadership:* Here the professional social group worker's role is to suggest, support, and encourage the cardiac support group membership. The social group worker is inclined to work for change, education, and socialization, sympathetic listening, and sharing.
2. *Active-participant leadership:* Here the professional social group worker's role is to provide direct leadership. The social group worker is in a prone position to facilitate goals of parent leaders and may focus more on medical or nursing interventions; empathetic listening and reflecting feelings can clarify misconceptions about cardiac care and potential outcomes based on lifestyle adjustments.

The professional social group worker's leadership needs depend on the group model. After selecting a group model based on the identified support needs and goals, it is important to determine the professional activities to be undertaken. A universal action that the professional can render in a nonintrusive manner is to share his or her knowledge about group process. The professional leader must be able to monitor and direct group participants, encourage expression of experiences, encourage sharing of coping strategies, refer to appropriate resources, emphasize responsibility, maintain positive attitudes toward challenges to make coping easier, actively listen, and minimize leader-dominated discussion.

CLINICAL TECHNIQUES UTILIZED

Irrespective of whether the cardiac support group is formal or informal, the core techniques that the social group should lend are direction, or redirection when appropriate, to help maintain a prosocial focus; instillation of hope, even in the most critical of cardiac cases; help dispel myths and misinformation (e.g., cardiac procedures, medication compliance issues, general course, and outcome of specific cardiovascular diseases, etc.) among members; maintain a sense of structure and order; and act as a proactive resource person. Beyond the professional understanding of group dynamics, the social group worker needs to be able to impart this information in a nonintrusive manner to support the group's integrity.

In addition, the social group worker will have to have specialized knowledge of the specific cardiovascular disease for which the support group was formed in order to serve as a responsible resource person. The social group worker should also facilitate the venting of thoughts (both positive and negative cognitions), feelings (both positive and negative affective expressions), concerns, and fears. Ventilation allows cardiac support group members a method that focuses on discharge of tension by airing feelings and problems. For ventilation to be therapeutic for the group-as-a-whole, the social group worker needs to ensure that these meetings do not turn into "gripe sessions" in which, by definition, there is little hope and lots of despair. Furthermore, the typical social group worker's leadership responsibilities will include the following: helping shape and direct the initial cardiac support group vision, spirit, and dedication; when feasible, organizing and conducting the initial cardiac support meetings so as to provide an appropriate, healthy, and prosocial role model; helping plan meetings with the members to determine the cardiac support group's aims, policies, and logistics; where possible, arranging for volunteers to share the group's administrative tasks. Delegate to and coordinate them, resolve conflicts in and among them, and recognize and appreciate them regularly for their efforts; conduct each cardiac support meeting effectively, or delegate that to another effective coleader. Set each meeting's tone (e.g., optimism versus gloom) and agenda, and follow it—unless unexpected crises arise.

Balance cardiac support group meetings' content dynamically between patients, their respective family members, and group operational tasks. Here, *effective* means that most of those attending the meetings get their major needs met in a way that everyone feels good about it.

Act as community spokesperson for the group (a macro role function for the social group worker), or delegate that job and monitor it. Stay aware of general and special cardiac support group needs, and coordinate the talents and resources of group members and the community to meet them. Balance individual cardiac patient needs with all group members' needs. Avoid overusing the group as a personal resource.

Make clear, timely administrative decisions about cardiac support group process. Confront problems promptly and assertively, which aids with prosocial modeling. Facilitate group problem solving supportively, when members conflict.

Negotiate with any guest speakers, and coordinate their time, focus, and participation. Monitor what cardiac support group members attend for, and whether they're getting enough of their needs met. If not, take responsibility for problem solving and reequilibrate the focus and purpose. Take (or delegate) overall responsibility for recruiting appropriate new members, and do so. Also ask for help with these responsibilities, and delegate, when they feel too much. Because this is asking a lot of one professional social group worker, having co-leadership can prevent burnout, illness, and responsibilities "falling through the cracks."

EXPECTED CLINICAL BENEFITS AND OUTCOMES

The most hopeful outcome of participation in a cardiac support group is that the members will gain some support, affiliation, and identification, and also develop a sense of hope. By affiliating with cardiac patients dealing with similar medical and psychosocial issues, members gain not only identification with fellow members, but are able to discern where they are relative to others. That is not to say that members' attendance and ultimate comparison with those who perceptually are at a less healthy place in terms of their cardiac disease will enhance their survival hope and rate, but by participation in the cardiac support group, it will give members a point in time to reference where they are concerning cardiovascular medical and psychosocial functions of fellow members. The self-help group helps to empower members and decrease feeling of victimization (Adamsen 2002).

CONCLUSIONS

Often, the term *support group* is threatening if it is viewed as therapy or an indication that the families need help. For some people, self-reliance, not mutual help, is essential for coping. For others, open expression of feelings in a group setting is difficult, but one-to-one support is helpful. By utilizing cardiac support groups, cardiac patients and family members are able to exert some control and direction over the process while having a professional social group worker present to provide operational direction, help, and oversight concerning maintaining the purpose, function, structure, and integrity of the group-as-a-whole. Individuals diagnosed with cardiovascular disease are afforded mutual aid and professional support by involvement in a social support group experience.

Chapter 15

Cardiac Social Groups
and Coleadership

INTRODUCTION

In conducting social work groups, coleadership invariably becomes a crucial issue. This particularly is true when the social group is complex and related to major medical conditions such as cardiovascular disease. In deciding the utilitarian use of coleadership, the decision should not be made based solely on personal attributes or the degree of comfort one might experience in leading with another, but rather on what would maximize the value to the group. Notwithstanding the obvious need of coleaders' need to establish a clinical working relationship based on trust, mutual professional respect, cooperation, and support, the professional relationship is one that should be integrative and team-oriented. Coleadership is not a simple process. It is a complex process in which each group worker needs to develop a working relationship, such that one can focus on the group process and the members instead of each other. Therefore, it is essential that coleaders meet frequently to discuss their differences and their views on the members in the group, the agreed upon group goals, and the management of the group process.

CARDIAC COLEADERSHIP: BACKGROUND

Leading social groups with one or more colleagues can be extremely advantageous, especially for the novice social group worker.

Social Group Work with Cardiac Patients
© 2007 by The Haworth Press, Inc. All rights reserved.
doi:10.1300/5739_15

Historically, social group work coleadership is a unique aspect that offers different perspective to the group-as-a-whole process (Rosenbaum 1971). It has traditionally been a responsible way to introduce group work to trainees (Donohue 2002). Social group work is also useful to seasoned social group workers. They can learn new therapeutic techniques by joining other social group workers to learn their style or techniques, or can have a visiting therapist for a few sessions in their ongoing group or a specially designed marathon (Eliot 1990).

Social group work coleadership is a professionally intimate relationship. The two social group workers come to know each other's personality, professional strengths, and assets, as well as the other's weaknesses and liabilities. They confront and support each other and resolve differences between themselves when possible. Social group work can offer their professional relationships as a problem-solving model to the group-as-a-whole, but their openness in discussing and dealing with problems between them must be carefully timed and dosed. Early in the development of the social cardiac group-as-a-whole, it is best that they work out professional disagreements in private, lest the overt tension between them disrupts the group. After the group has developed, the ability to tolerate, deal, and manage coleadership, problems can be occasionally introduced in the social group by mutual agreement of the social group coleaders, when they feel that a specific purpose can be addressed.

ADVANTAGES OF COLEADERSHIP

One major advantage is that it is quite often easier than leading a group alone. The involvement of oneself with a coleader can be a very valuable tool for both training and helping maximize the overall group work process. A coleader can provide support and relief for another, especially when working with the intensity of cardiac groups in general, and specifically, if one leader gets professionally stuck or emotionally drained. In addition, coleadership can provide additional ideas for planning the social group and can share the responsibility for leading during the session. Coleadership often brings different viewpoints, perspectives, and varied life experiences to the group-as a-whole, providing members with alternative sources of opinion and information on a specific cardiac topical area. Differences in the interpersonal style of each coleader can also serve and create variations in the process group flow or the overall tenor of the group, thereby making the group work experience more interesting and meaningful to the cardiac patient members. There may also be occasions when a coleader with more specialized knowledge about a given population is needed, as in the case of a topical cardiac social group that deals with nutrition, medications, and exercises that promote cardiac recovery.

Coleadership can also serve as models for cardiac members of the group. Effective interaction skills and cooperation are demonstrated by coleaders who work well together. Often opposite-sex coleaders may serve as role models and may be particularly effective in working with mixed gender groups, as well as in social group work with family members. In certain social groups, male and female teams can also serve as healthy parental figures for cardiac members who are from dysfunctional family-of-origins that have unresolved family issues. However, it is important to note that it is not essential that coleaders be of the opposite sex. Many social groups are led by coleaders of the same sex.

The final advantage of coleadership is that leaders get feedback from another leader. Furthermore, leaders learn from watching each other handle various situations. For maximal awareness of nonverbal cues, coleaders should sit across from each other in the social group circle (Jacobs, Masson, and Harvill 1998). According to Jacobs, Masson, and Harvill (1998), coleadership provides an opportunity for the members to easily maintain eye contact with one another while allowing observations of the cardiac social group members from different vantage points.

DISADVANTAGES OF COLEADERSHIP

There are several disadvantages of coleadership. One is that coleading takes time away from other counseling duties and can add stress to an already demanding workload and schedule. Therefore, coleading social group work with cardiac patients may not be a good use of staff's time and efforts.

Problems with coleadership with cardiac social groups arise mainly from differences in attitude, therapeutic style, and goals of the leaders. Coleading social groups becomes a disadvantage when the two leaders do not conceptualize the social group in a similar manner. As Corey and Corey (1977) note, the choice of a coleader is important. If two leaders are incompatible (on theoretical or personal grounds), their group is bound to be negatively affected. The leaders can confuse the social group members because they each want to direct the social group in a certain direction.

SOCIAL GROUP WORK COLEADERSHIP MODELS

There are two fundamental models of social group work coleadership. Each of these models assumes that the coleaders are committed to identifying, discussing, and developing goals for the group-as-a-whole, as well as for each session. The model utilized will depend on the overall purpose and goals of the social group, the experience of the two leaders, the individual styles of the coleaders, and the degree to which the coleaders feel they can negotiate and coordinate their efforts.

Alternating Leadership

This model is one in which coleaders alternate in taking the primary group worker role. Alternating roles are usually decided upon during the planning and formation of a group session. For example, one coleader may be responsible for one week's session in terms of attending to the content of the group, while the other group worker attends to the process elements of the group. Then depending on the session, the roles of each can be reversed. With exposure, experience, and time, the coleaders who work well together find that shifting of roles goes smoothly.

The alternating of coleadership may be appropriate if the coleaders differ somewhat in their approaches and find themselves pulling the social group in opposing directions. Alternating leadership allows one coleader to have primary responsibility for directing the group for a specific period of time without concern, relative to being interrupted by the other coleader. This does not imply that the second coleader is totally inactive. That is to say, the coleader may offer supporting comments, clarity, or summarize as appropriate to enhance the overall functioning of the group-as-a-whole.

Shared Leadership

The shared model of coleadership is one in which each leader shares the leadership in total, with neither designated as the primary leader during a specific time period. In this model, the group workers "flow" with one another and lead jointly. Thus, in this model both the group coleaders share in attending to the process and content of the group-as-whole. Although in this model the coleaders work together, at times, one leader will take charge, such as when conducting an exercise or working with an individual cardiac group member. Moreover, the other group leader is ready to take charge at any point and continue in the same therapeutic direction. This is particularly helpful if one or the other coleader gets stuck in a therapeutic rut and/or is not expert on a particular topic being addressed.

When using this shared coleadership model, social group workers should be careful not to echo each other's words or concepts. That is to say, one social group worker will say something, and then the other social group worker will say something that is very similar to the first leader's comments. Furthermore, it is paramount that the leaders not join in commenting on the other social group worker when the social group workers are interacting at the emotional expense and exclusion of the cardiac group members.

SELECTION OF A SOCIAL GROUP
WORK COLEADER

Coleadership is suggested using a male and a female social group worker for the conjoint treatment of most disorders to provide for health modeling and to enhance gender specific communications, especially when dealing with sexuality as a theme. One the other hand, there are people who will question the need for male-female coleadership, and to date, there is no clinical evidence that a mixed-sex cotherapy team has significant advantages over a like-sex pair. However, clinical practice wisdom seems to support coleadership in most forms of social work with groups. The most important qualities of coleaders are their ability to withstand the confrontations necessary for conflict resolution between them, and their agreement in attitudes toward working with cardiac patients in a social group context. Different personality types and professional differences between social group workers can be useful if they result in a complementary fashion (Starak 1982).

The professional qualifications of the social group workers are less important than their ability to work together. Often, prospective social group work coleaders need one or more preliminary conferences to discuss their theoretical orientations, their goals for the projected group, and their commitment to the goals and focus of the cardiac social group. Moreover, they can also explore each other's areas of difficulty in dealing with cardiac patients, and the areas in which each considers himself or herself to be strong. What each social group worker knows of his or her own style should also be shared. Irrespective of theoretical and practical differences, the social group work coleaders need to submit to oversight, joint supervision, and/or consultation on a regular basis.

MANAGING PROBLEMS THAT EMERGE
IN SOCIAL GROUP WORK COLEADERSHIP

General Issues and Problems Associated
with Social Group Coleadership

Competition for Authority Among Social Group Workers

When each social group leader wants to be in charge:
This can happen when each social group worker has a drastically different practice orientation (e.g., psychodynamic versus cognitive-behavioral), or when clarity has not been established between the social work group leaders. Ideally, coleaders should have met and discussed their clinical/practice orientation, their approach to cardiac recovery, and discussed any concerns, such as which coleadership model they plan to use and who will attend to process aspects versus content aspects of treatment.

Interpersonal Problems Among Social Group Workers

Social group workers may dislike one another personally or professionally, and this understandably can hinder successful treatment. Therefore, treatment is negatively affected.

Differing Approaches to Group Leadership

For example, one leader may prefer a group-as-a-whole perspective, whereas the other leader prefers to view the group as a collection of members in which individual therapy occurs.

If either or both social group leaders have a need to compete or dominate the group, coleading will be difficult, and the ones who suffer the most are the social group members. Theoretically, social group work coleaders should work together using a team approach. In clinical practice, the process of social group work coleadership should contribute to, rather than detract from, the overall group experience. Social group workers should be secure in their relative position in the group and must professionally respect each other so as to facilitate a healthy clinical working relationship.

When the two social group leaders have drastically different clinical styles of leading, or opposing views on how to proceed in the group-as-a-whole, coleadership is not recommended. Although clinical differences can be valuable, the diametric differences can potentially cause friction and frustration that the cardiac group members most likely will perceive. For example, if one of the social group members was trained to focus mostly on process and the other to focus mostly on content, each leader would be frustrated by the other's style of leadership.

A further component of social group work coleadership is that the leaders should be willing to set aside time to plan each session and share feedback and concerns. The overall advantage of social group work coleadership breaks down if either of the coleaders is unwilling to take necessary time to plan, actuate the group, compromise, and negotiate. Practice wisdom suggests that social group coleaders who try to go to the group meetings without having prepared jointly, risk having a group that is not dynamically fluid (process integration). This may lead to conflict and disruption between the coleaders. In essence, social group work coleadership requires the joint commitment of the group workers working together for the overall benefit of the cardiac group members.

USE OF SOCIAL GROUP WORK COLEADERSHIP WITH CARDIAC PATIENTS

For most social groups developed for cardiac patients, the use of coleaders is strongly recommended. The rationale is that much of what occurs in cardiac social groups has a technical aspect that requires at least one of the leaders to have specialized knowledge. For example, many cardiac social groups such as nutritional, stress management, anger management, and cardiac treatment compliance each require a sophisticated knowledge base. Ideally, both coleaders would have this knowledge base, but in real situations, there needs to be at least one of the leaders thus trained.

In cardiac social groups that are not so technical, the use of a coleader is preferred because of the intense emotionality of these groups. Therapy groups, such as an interpersonal social group, require a high level of process attention. In addition, a single social group worker often cannot monitor the totality of overt and covert messaging and emotionality that occurs in cardiac social groups dealing with potentially life-threatening diseases.

For similar reasons (i.e., the technical and emotionally intense nature of cardiac social groups), leading these groups can be intellectually and emotionally taxing on group workers. By having a coleader, the group worker can gain needed intellectual and emotional support. Also, having a coleader in cardiac social group work allows for a natural check-and-balance relative to preparing for sessions, monitoring for misinformation, and processing recent session relative to group outcome (success versus failure of the group in meeting the group-as-a-whole goals and the current sessions goals), and group output (i.e., what actually happened in the course of the social group session).

CONCLUSIONS

The psychosocial treatment of individuals diagnosed with cardiovascular disease is extremely complex. Therefore, the psychosocial treatment of cardiac patients invariably becomes more complex. The use of a group work coleader is frequently necessary, given the complexity of the focus and purpose of the social group. Hence, the social group worker needs to know his or her limitations relative to the purpose of the cardiac social group. It is wise to have coleaders involved in topical or specialized cardiac areas that are complex and in which the social group worker may not have the requisite knowledge.

If a coleader is deemed as needed, given the topic and purpose of the social group to be dealt with, it is strongly suggested that the social group worker treating cardiac patients meet with the coleader in advance of the first session to address the following:

- The role that each coleader will play within the cardiac social group
- The theoretical orientation of both coleaders
- Ways in which the coleaders will manage variance and conflicts
- An agreement that the coleaders will process each group session to discern ways to improve the cardiac social group
- Clinical triggers that indicate that the coleaders need to consult with an outside professional when conflict is assessed as not resolvable

The prudent social group worker will monitor the cardiac group and humble himself or herself to seek help as needed.

Chapter 16

Conclusions:
Integration of Social Group Work
with Cardiac Patients

Working with cardiac patients is challenging and complex. For the social group worker to be effective, he or she needs a comprehensive understanding of cardiovascular disease, a working knowledge of social group work techniques and content, and an understanding of the potential process outcomes, based on both traditional and current models of social group work. The beginner social group workers will need oversight and consistent supervision while an advance social group worker would benefit from ongoing consultation.

Much of the social group work will inevitably be linked to involvement with cardiac patients and their respective family members, since the development of cardiac patients affects the entire family. Therefore, more specific intervention will need to be developed for family members as they grapple with the biopsychosocial complexities inherent in having a family member diagnosed with a cardiovascular disease.

This book serves the purpose of helping the beginner social group worker develop fundamental skills in the utilization of group process and group techniques. Also, the book has served the purpose of advancing therapy skills in more advanced social work clinicians. The book has been an attempt to inform both the beginner and more seasoned social group workers on the purpose, function, structure, and expected outcomes for cardiac social groups in general group contexts and in specific group types.

Social Group Work with Cardiac Patients
© 2007 by The Haworth Press, Inc. All rights reserved.
doi:10.1300/5739_16

The overall approach here was to enhance the social group workers' knowledge base and their understanding of fundamental state-of-the-art cardiac psychosocial care. The social work groups highlighted in this book were chosen based on the comprehensive psychosocial needs of cardiac patients.

Many of the cardiac social groups are complex relative to topic and technical involvement. The prudent social group worker will seek oversight, supervision, and consultations as needed. Truly, the psychosocial and medical treatment of cardiovascular patients is an interdisciplinary process. Owing to the myriad technical and emotional issues associated with dealing with the psychosocial aspects of cardiac disease, there is a professional need for collaboration in the treatment of cardiac patients in a social group in an interdisciplinary manner (i.e., the use of several disciplinary perspectives in tandem) rather than a multidisciplinary manner (i.e., where professionals from various disciplines interact and work with the cardiac patient in discrete, but separate manners). Given the complexity of leading cardiac social groups, in most instances, the social group worker should enlist the help of a coleader who has specialized knowledge and skills in the specific topical area.

Furthermore, this book has been an attempt to synthesize social, psychological, and biologic factors of cardiovascular disease with the fundamental and complex practice of social group work. The degree to which the social group worker can successfully integrate the state-of-the-art understanding of cardiac disease with the current practice of social group work will enhance the effectiveness of the social group worker as well as, provide the cardiac patient with the most current cardiac information and social group work interventions. There remains an unmet need in the area of social work research concerning the efficaciousness of group models in general, and there is a specific gap in the available research on chronic biopsychosocial problems such as cardiovascular disease. Social group workers and social work researchers will need to invest in academic resources in understanding what social groups work best with specific cardiac patients and how these groups work. By beginning with the premise that social groups can potentially help cardiac patients, and expected outcomes for cardiac patients are realistic, social work researchers will be able to gain a more comprehensive understanding of how social groups effect positive change.

Although not dealt with in this book, the use of family therapy as a special form of social group work needs to be researched relative to how family members grapple with cardiac disease, what expectations the family of a cardiac patient have, and the ways in which family members and significant others adapt are paramount to cardiovascular illness is addressed. Finally, social work research needs to address the concept of coping with the death of cardiac patients. This is particularly important when the cardiac patient is a child with a congenital cardiovascular disease. Although the death of a loved one is typically difficult, the death of a child diagnosed with a cardiovascular disease is particularly complex in that it can be sudden or protracted depending on whether the heart problems are congenital versus developmental in nature. That is to say, families who have a cardiac patient who has a congenital cardiac disease have a different frame of reference than those who develop a cardiac disease in early childhood, adolescence, or an unexpected death (e.g., a minor child who dies from cardiovascular disease that heretofore has not been medically detected).

Bibliography

Adamsen, L. (2002). "From victim to agent": The clinical and social significance of self-help group participation for people with life-threatening diseases. *Scandinavian Journal of Caring Sciences*, 16(3): 224-232.

Adamsen, J. and Rasmussen, J. (2001). Sociological perspective on self-help groups: Reflections on conceptualization and social processes. *Journal of Advance Nursing*, 35(6): 909-917.

Agency for Healthcare Research and Quality (2000). Addressing racial and ethnic disparities in health care. Fact Sheet. AHRQ Publication No. 00-P041. *Agency for Healthcare Research and Quality*, Rockville, MD. http://www.ahrq.gov/research/disparit.htm.

Alexander, J. and Parsons, B. (2000). Short-term family intervention: A therapy outcome study. *Journal of Counseling and Clinical Psychology*, 2: 195-201.

Alexander, J. and Robins, M. (1999). Family therapy with older, indicated youth: From promise to proof to practice. In K. Kumpfer (Ed.). *Center for Substance Abuse Prevention Science Symposium: Bridging the Gap Between Research and Practice*. Washington, DC: Center for Substance Abuse and Prevention.

Alexander, J., Sexton, T., and Robbins, M. (2000). The developmental status of family therapy in family intervention science. In H. Liddle, D. Santisteban, R. Leavant, and J. Bray (Eds.). *Family Psychology Intervention Science*. Washington, DC: American Psychological Association Press.

American College of Cardiology/American Heart Association (2005) Task force on performance measures for adults with heart failure. *Journal of the American College of Cardiology* 46(6): 1144-1178.

American Heart Association (AHA) Task Force on Risk Reduction (1998). Primary prevention of coronary heart disease: Guidance from Framingham. *Circulation*, 97: 1876-1887.

American Heart Association (AHA) (2005a). African Americans and Cardiovascular Diseases—Statistics. Dallas, TX: *American Heart Association Publications*.

American Heart Association (AHA) (2005b). Cardiovascular health disparities must be eradicated. Dallas, TX: *American Heart Association Publications*.

American Psychiatric Association (2000). Diagnostic and statistical manual of mental disorders, fourth edition, text revision (DSM-IV-TR). Arlington, VA: *American Psychiatric Association Press*.

Asilonlu, K. and Celik, S. (2004). The effects of preoperative education on anxiety of open cardiac surgery patients. *Patient Educational Counseling*, 53(1): 65-70.

Ausbrooks, E., Thomas, S., and Williams, R. (1995). Relationships among self-effi-cacy, optimism, trait anger, and anger expression. *Health Values, 19*(4): 46-53.

Bandura, A. (1973). *Aggression: A social learning analysis.* Englewood Cliffs, NJ: Prentice-Hall.

Barker, R. (1999). *The social work dictionary* (4th ed.). Silver Springs, MD: NASW Press.

Bax, J., Abraham, T., Barold, S. S., Breithardt, O. A., Fung, J. W. H., Garrigue, S., Gorcsan, J. III, Hayes, D. L., Kass, D. A., Knuuti, J., Leclercq, C., Linde, C., Mark, D. B., Monaghan, M. J., Nihoyannopoulos, P., Schalij, M. J., Stellbrink, C., and Yu, C. M. (2005a). Cardiac resynchronization therapy: Part 1: Issues before device implantation. *The Journal of American College of Cardiology,* 46: 2153-2167.

Bax, J., Abraham, T., Barold, S. S., Breithardt, O. A., Fung, J. W. H., Garrigue, S., Gorcsan, J. III, Hayes, D. L., Kass, D. A., Knuuti, J., Leclercq, C., Linde, C., Mark, D. B., Monaghan, M. J., Nihoyannopoulos, P., Schalij, M. J., Stellbrink, C., and Yu, C. M. (2005b). Cardiac resynchronization therapy: Part 2: Issues during and after device implantation and unresolved questions. *The Journal of American College of Cardiology,* 46: 2168-2182.

Beck, A. and Emery, G. (1985). *Anxiety disorder and phobia: A cognitive perspective.* New York: Basic Books.

Beck, A., Rush, A., Shaw, B., and Emery, G. (1979). *Cognitive therapy of depression.* New York: Guilford Press.

Beck, J. (1995). *Cognitive therapy: Basic and beyond.* New York: Guilford Press.

Becker, M. (1976). The health belief model and personal health behavior. *Health Education Monographs,* 2(4): 324-473.

Betz, C., Unger, O., Frager, B., Test, L., and Smith, C. (1990). A survey of self-help groups in California for parents of children with chronic conditions. *Pediatric Nursing,* 16: 293-296.

Blumenthal, J., Jiang, W., Babyak, M., Krantz, D., Frid, D., Coleman, R., Waugh, R., Hanson, M., Appelbaum, M., O'Connor, C., and Morris, J. (1997). Stress management and exercise training in cardiac patients with myocardial ischemia: Effects on prognosis and evaluation of mechanisms. *Archives of Internal Medicine,* 157: 2213-2223.

Blumenthal, A., Jiang, W., Waugh, R., Frid, D., Morris, J., Coleman, R. Hanson, M., Babyak, M., Thyrum, E., Krantz, D., and O'Connor, C. (1995). Mental stress-induced ischemia in the laboratory and ambulatory ischemia during daily life. *Circulation,* 92: 2102-2108.

Bosworth, H., Siegler, I., Brummmett, B., Barfefoot, J., Williams, R., Channing, N., and Mark, D. (1999). The association between self-rated health and mortality in a well-characterized sample or coronary artery disease patients. *Medical Care,* 37(12): 1226-1236.

Brabender, V. and Fallon, A. (1993). *Models of group psychotherapy.* Washington, DC: American Psychiatric Association.

Brackett, D., Gauvin, D., and Lerner, M. (1994). Cardiovascular responses induced by ethanol. *The Journal of Pharmacology and Experimental Therapeutics,* 268: 78-84.

Bradley, K. and Williams, D. (1990). A comparison of the preoperative concerns of open heart surgery patients and their significant others. *Journal of Cardiovascular Nursing*, 5(1): 43-53.

Bricker, D. and Young, J. (1993). *A client's guide to schema-focused cognitive therapy*. New York: Cognitive Therapy Center.

Brook, D. (2005). Exploring group therapies. *Psychiatric Times*, XX (2).

Brook, J., Rosen, Z., and Brook, D. (2001).The effect of early marijuana use on later anxiety and depressive symptoms. *NYS Psychologist*, 35-39.

Brown, D., Glazer, H., and Higgins, M. (1983). Group intervention: A psychosocial and educational approach to open heart surgery patients and their families. *Social Work in Health Care*, 9(2): 47-59.

Budaj, A., Flasinska, K., Gore, J., Anderson, F., Jr, Dabbous, O., Spencer, F., Goldberg, R., and Fox, K. (2005). Magnitude of and risk factors for in-hospital and postdischarge stroke in patients with acute coronary syndromes findings from a global registry of acute coronary events. *Circulation*, 111: 3242-3247.

Burg, M. and Abrams, D. (2001). Depression in chronic medical illness: The case of coronary heart disease. *Journal of Clinical Psychology*, 57(11): 1323-1337.

Burns, D. (1999). *The feeling good handbook: The new mood therapy*. New York: Penguin.

Burns, S. and Burns, K. (1990). *How to survive unbearable stress* (2nd ed.). Revised for electronic distribution: http://www.teachhealth.com.

Byrne, D. and Kelley, K. (1981). *An introduction to personality* (3rd ed.). Englewood Cliffs, NJ: Prentice Hall.

Carney, R., Freedland, K., Miller, G., and Jaffe, A. (2002). Depression as a risk factor for cardiac mortality and morbidity: A review of potential mechanisms. *Journal of Psychosomatic Research*, 53(4): 897-902.

Center for Substance Abuse Treatment (2004). *Substance abuse treatment and family therapy*. Treatment Improvement Protocol (TIP) Series, No. 39, DHHS Publication No. (SMA) 05-4006. Rockville, MD: Substance Abuse and Mental Health Services Administration.

Center for Substance Abuse Treatment (2005). *Substance abuse treatment: Group therapy*. Treatment Improvement Protocol (TIP) Series, No. 41, DHHS Publication No. (SMA) 05-4006. Rockville, MD: Substance Abuse and Mental Health Services Administration.

Centers for Disease Control and Prevention (CDC) (1983). Perspectives in disease prevention and health promotion alcohol as a risk factor for injuries—United States. *Morbidly Mortally Weekly Report*, 32(5): 61-62.

Centers for Disease Control and Prevention (2004). Disparities in premature deaths from heart disease: 50 states and the District of Columbia, 2001. *Morbidly Mortally Weekly Report*, 53: 121-125.

Centers for Disease Control and Prevention (CDC) (2005a). *First national health and nutrition examination survey (NHANES I) public use data files*. Hayattsville, MD: U.S. Department of Health and Human Services, National Center for Health Statistics.

Centers for Disease Control and Prevention (CDC) (2005b). Racial/ethnic and socioeconomic disparities in multiple risk factors for heart disease and stroke: United States, 2003. *Morbidly Mortally Weekly Report*, 54: 113-117.

Centers for Disease Control and Prevention (CDC) (2005). *Vital health statistics 10.* No. 225. Hayattsville, MD: U.S. Department of Health and Human Services, National Center for Health Statistics.

Champion, V. (1984). Instrument development for health belief model constructs. *Advances in Nursing Science,* 6: 73-85.

Chang, P., Ford, D., Meoni, L., Wang, N., and Klag, M. (2002). Anger in young men and subsequent premature cardiovascular disease: The precursors study. *Archives of Internal Medicine* 22; 162(8): 901-906.

Chapman, D.P., Perry, G., and Strine, T. (2005). The vital link between chronic disease and depressive disorders. *Prev Chronic Dis* [serial online]. Jan [date cited]. Available from: URL: http://www.cdc.gov/pcd/issues/2005/jan/04_0066.htm.

Corey, G. and Corey, M. (1977). *Groups: Process and practice.* Monterey, CA: Brooks/Cole.

Corti, R., Binggeli, C., and Sudano, I. (2002). Coffee acutely increases sympathetic nerve activity and blood pressure independently of caffeine content: Role of habitual versus nonhabitual drinking. *Circulation,* 106: 2935-2940.

Coward, D. (1990). Critical multiplism: A research strategy for nursing science. *Image: Journal of Nursing Scholarship,* 22: 163-167.

Crone, C. and Wise, T. (1999). Psychiatric aspects of transplantation. I: Evaluation and selection of candidates. *Critical Care Nursing,* 19: 79-87.

Dattilio, F. and Freeman, A. (Eds.). (1994). *Cognitive-behavioral strategies in crisis intervention* (2nd ed.). New York: Guilford.

Davies, N. (2000a). Carers' opinions and emotional responses following cardiac surgery: Cardiac rehabilitation implications for critical care nurses. *Intensive Critical Care Nursing,* 16(2): 66-75.

Davies, N. (2000b). Patients' and carers' perceptions of factors influences recovery after cardiac surgery. *Journal of Advance Nursing,* 32(2): 318-326.

Daviglus, M., Stamler, J., Pirzada, A., Yan, L., Garside, D., Liu, K., Wang, R., Dyer, A., Lloyd-Jones, D., and Greenland, P. (2004). Favorable cardiovascular risk profile in young women and long-term risk of cardiovascular and all-cause mortality. *The Journal of American Medical Association,* 292: 1588-1592.

Deffenbacher, J. (1995). Ideal treatment package for adults with anger. In H. Kassinove (Ed.), *Anger Disorders: Definition, Diagnosis, and Treatment.* (pp. 151-172). Washington, DC: Taylor & Francis.

Denollet, J. and Brutsaert, D. (1998). Personality, disease severity, and the risk of long-term cardiac events in patients with a decreased ejection fraction after myocardial infarction. *Circulation,* 97: 167-173.

Dies, R. (1992a). The future of group psychotherapy. *Psychotherapy,* 29(1): 58-64.

Dies, R. (1992b). Models of group psychotherapy: Sifting through the confusion. *International Journal of Group Psychotherapy,* 42(1): 1-17.

Donohue, M. (2002). Group coleadership by occupational therapy students in community centers: Learning transitional roles. *Occupational Therapy in Health Care,* 15(1/2): 85-98.

Droppleman, P. and Witt, D. (1993). Women, depression, and anger. In S.P. Thomas (Ed.), *Women and Anger* (pp. 209-232). New York: Springer.

Duits, A., Duivenvoorden, H., and Boeke, S. (1998) The course of anxiety and depression in patients undergoing coronary artery bypass graft surgery. *Journal of Psychosomatic Research*, 45(2): 127-138.

Dunlap, K. (1996). Functional theory and social work practice. In F. Turner (Ed.). *Social Work Treatment*, (4th ed.) (pp. 319-340). New York: The Free Press.

Eisen, M. (1992). A health belief model—Social learning theory approach to adolescents' fertility control: Findings from a controlled field trial. *Health Education Quarterly*, 19: 249-262.

Eliot, A. (1990). Group coleadership: A new role for parents of adolescents with anorexia and bulimia nervosa. *International Journal of Group Psychotherapy*, 40(3): 339-351.

Ellen, E. (1999). Group therapy requires good clinical judgment, careful screening. *Psychiatric Times*, XVI(10): 3-5.

Ellis, T. and Newman, C.F. (1996). *Choosing to live: How to defeat suicide through cognitive therapy.* Oakland, CA: New Harbinger.

Fallon, J., Keator, D., Mbogori, J., Turner, J., and Potkin, S. (2004). Hostility differentiates the brain metabolic effects of nicotine. *Cognitive Brain Research*, 18(2): 142-148.

Faupel, A., Herrick, E., and Sharp, P. (1998). *Anger management: A practical guide.* New York: David Fulton Publications.

Feeny, N., Zoeliner, L., and Fitzgibbons, L. (2000). Exploring the roles of emotional numbing, depression, and discussion in PTSD. *Journal of Traumatic Stress*, 13(3): 489-498.

Feign, R., Cohen, I., and Gilad, M. (1998). The use of single-group sessions in discharge planning. *Social Work in Health Care*, 26(3): 19-38.

Festinger, L. (1957). *A theory of cognitive dissonance.* Stanford, CA: Stanford University Press.

Fisher, M. (1995). Group therapy protocols for persons with a personality disorder who abuse substances: Effective treatment alternatives. *Social Work with Groups*, 18(4): 71-89.

Fisher, M. (2004). Group for substance abuse treatment. In C. Garvin, L. Gutierrez, and M. Galinsky (Eds.), *Handbook of Social Work Groups* (pp. 259-274). New York: Guilford Press.

Fisher, M. and Bentley, K. (1996). Effectiveness study of two group therapy models with dually diagnosed consumers. *Psychiatric Services*, 47(11): 1244-1250.

Flores, P. (1997). *Group psychotherapy with addicted populations.* Binghamton, NY: Haworth Press.

Ford, E., Giles, W., and Mokdad, A. (2004). The distribution of 10-year risk for coronary heart disease among US adults: Findings from the National Health and Nutrition Survey III. *Journal of American College of Cardiology* 43: 1791-1796.

Fox, C., Evans, J., Larson, M., Kannel, W., and Levy, D. (2004). Temporal trends in coronary heart disease mortality and sudden cardiac death from 1950-1999: The Framingham Heart Study. *Circulation*, 110: 522-527.

Frasure-Smith, N., Lesperance, F., and Talajic, M. (1995). Depression and 18-month prognosis after myocardial infarction. *Circulation*, 91(4): 999-1005.

Freeman, A. and Dattilio, F. (Eds.). (1992). *Comprehensive casebook of cognitive therapy.* New York: Plenum Press.

Freeman, A., Pretzer, J., Fleming, B., and Simon, K. (1990). *Clinical applications of cognitive therapy.* New York: Plenum Press.

Garrison, R., Feinleib, M., Castelli, W., and McNamara, P. (1983). Cigarette smoking as a confounder of the relationship between relative weight and long-term mortality: The Framingham Heart Study. *The Journal of American Medical Association,* 249: 2199-2203.

Getzel, G. (2004). Groups in physical and mental health. In C. Garvin, L. Gutierrez, and M. Galinsky (Eds.), *Handbook of Social Work Groups* (pp. 195-211). New York: Guilford Press.

Gier, M., Levick, N., and Blazina, P. (1988). Stress reduction with heart transplant patients and their families: A multidisciplinary approach. *Journal of Heart Transplant,* 7(5): 342-347.

Gillis, C., Neuhaus, J., and Hauck, W. (1990). Improving family functioning after cardiac surgery: A randomized trial. *Heart and Lung,* 19(6): 648-654.

Gitterman, A. (2004). The mutual aid model. In C. Garvin, L. Gutierrez, and M. Galinsky (Eds.), *Handbook of Social Work Groups* (pp. 93-110). New York: Guilford Press.

Glasser, W. (1998). *Choice theory: A new psychology of personal freedom.* New York: Harper Paperbacks.

Goleman, D. (1995). *Emotional intelligence.* New York: Bantam.

Gottieb, B. (1982). Mutual-help groups: Members' views of their family benefits and the role for professionals. *Preventative Human Services,* 1(3): 55-67.

Grace, S., Hershenfield, K., Robertson, E., and Stewart, D.E. (2004). Factors affecting perceived risk of contracting severe acute respiratory syndrome among academic physicians. *Infection Control and Hospital Epidemiology,* 25(12): 1111-1113.

Grady, K., Jalowicc, A., and White-Williams, C. (1999). Preoperative psychosocial predictors of hospital length of stay for heart transplantation. *Journal of Cardiovascular Nursing,* 14(1): 12-26.

Greenberg, D. and Padesky, C. (1995). *Mind over mood: A cognitive therapy treatment manual for clients.* New York: Guilford.

Greenlund, K., Keenan, N., Giles, W., Zheng, Z., Neff, L., Croft, J., and Mensah, G. (2004). Public recognition of major signs and symptoms of heart attack: Seventeen states and the US Virgin Islands, 2001. *American Heart Journal,* 147: 1010-1016.

Groves, J. (1978). Taking care of the hateful patient. *New England Journal of Medicine,* 298: 883-887.

Haley, J. (1990). *Strategies of psychotherapy.* New York: Triangle Press/W.W. Norton & Company.

Haley, J. (1991). *Problem-solving therapy.* San Francisco: Jossey-Bass Publishers.

Hamilton, G. (1940). *Theory and Practice of Casework.* New York: Columbia University Press.

Hamilton, G. and Seidman, R. (1993). A comparison of the recovery period for women and men after an acute myocardial infarction. *Heart Lung,* 22(4): 308-315.

Hathaway, D., Combs, C., De Geest, S., Stergachis, A., and Moore, L. (1999). Patient compliance in transplantation: A report on the perceptions of transplant clinicians. *Transplantation Proceedings*, 31(suppl 4A): 10S-13S.

Hawton, K., Salkovskis, P., Kirk, J., and Clark, D. (1989). *Cognitive behaviour therapy for psychiatric problems: A practical guide.* Oxford: Oxford University Press.

Health Care Financing Review (2004). *Medicare and Medicaid statistical supplement.* Baltimore, Maryland: U.S. Department of Health and Human Services.

Heimberger, R. and Becker, R. (2002). *Cognitive-behavioral group therapy for social phobias: Basic mechanism and clinical strategies.* New York: Guilford Press.

Heitkamp, H. and Scheib, K. (1991). Long-term results of group therapy in heart patients: A retrospective analysis. *Fortschr Medicine*, 109(35): 713-716. German Trans.

Hildingh, C. and Fridlund, B. (2003). Participation in peer support groups after a cardiac event: A 12-month follow-up. *Rehabilitation Nursing*, 28(4): 123-128.

Hildingh, C., Segesten, K., Bengtsson, C., and Fridlund, B. (1994). Experiences of socialsupport among participants in self-help groups related to coronary heart disease. *Journal of Clinical Nursing*, 3(4): 219-226.

Hoffman, L. (1981). *Foundations of family therapy.* New York: Basic Books, Inc., Publishers.

Hubert, H., Holford, T., and Kannel, W. (1982). Clinical characteristics and cigarette smoking in relation to prognosis of angina pectoris in Framingham. *American Journal of Epidemiology*, 115: 231-242.

Hurst, W. (2002). *The heart, arteries, and veins* (10th ed.). New York, NY: McGraw-Hill.

Hutchinson, G. and Chapman, B. (2005). Logotherapy-Enhanced REBT: An integration of discovery and reason. *Journal of Contemporary Psychotherapy*, 35(2): 145-155.

Hyler, B., Corley, M., and McMahon, D. (1985). The role of nursing in a support group for heart transplantation recipients and their families. *Journal of Heart Transplantation*, 4(4): 453-456.

Jacobs, E., Masson, R., and Harville, R. (1998). *Group counseling: Strategies and skills.* New York: Brooks/Cole Publishing.

Jiang, W. and Davidson, J. (2005). Antidepressant therapy in patients with ischemic heart disease. *American Heart Journal*, 150(5): 871-881.

Johnston, L., O'Malley, P., and Bachman, J. (2005). *Monitoring the future; National results on adolescent drug use, overview and key findings, 2004.* NIH Pub. No. 05-5506. Bethesda, MD: NIDA, NIH, DHHS.

Kahn, E. (1996). Coleadership: Gender issues in group psychotherapy. In B. DeChant (Ed.), *Women and Gtroup Psychotherapy: Theory and Practice.* (pp. 442-462) New York: Guildford Press.

Kannel, W. (1978). Hypertension, blood lipids, and cigarette smoking as co-risk factors for coronary heart disease. *Annals of the New York Academy of Sciences*, 304: 128-139.

Kannel, W. (1988). Contributions of the Framingham Study to the conquest of coronary artery disease. *American Journal of Cardiology*, 62: 1109-1112.

Kannel, W., Hjortland, M., McNamara, P., and Gordon, T. (1976). Menopause and risk of cardiovascular disease: The Framingham study. *Annals of Internal Medicine*, 85: 447-452.

Kaplan, B. and Sadock, S. (2004). *Comprehensive textbook of psychiatry*. New York: Lippincott Williams & Wilkins.

Kaplan, H., Sadock, B., and Grebb, J. (1994). *Kaplan and Sadock's synopsis of psychiatry: Behavioral sciences, clinical psychiatry*. New York: Lippincott Williams & Wilkins.

Katz, A. and Bender, E. (1976). *The strength in us: Self-help in the modern world*. New York: Franklin Watts Press.

Kech, M. and Buddle, B. (1999). Ambulatory heart groups after inpatient cardiologic rehabilitation. *Rehabilitation*, 38(2): 79-87.

Kim, J. (2003). Caffeine and coffee tolerance. *Circulation*, 108: e38.

King, K. and Gortner, S. (1996). Women's short-term recovery from cardiac surgery. *Progressive Cardiovascular Nursing*, 11(2): 5-15.

King, K. and Jensen, L. (1994). Preserving the self: Women having cardiac surgery. *Heart and Lung*, 23(2): 99-105.

Kloner, R. (2004). Cardiovascular effects of the 3 phosphodiesterase-5 inhibitors approved for the treatment of erectile dysfunction. *Circulation*, 110(19): 3149-3155.

Kohm, C., Pollinger, D., and Sheriff, F. (2000). Creating cost-efficient initiatives in social work practice in the cardiac program of an acute care hospital. *Health and Social Work*, 25(2): 149-152.

Kubler-Ross, E. (1969). *On death and dying*. New York: Simon & Schuster/Touchstone.

Kubler-Ross, E. (1972). *Questions & answers on death and dying*. New York: Simon & Schuster/Touchstone.

Kubler-Ross, E. (1997). *The wheel of life*. New York: Simon & Schuster/Scribner.

Kuehlwein, K. and Rosen, H. (Eds.). (1993). *Cognitive therapies in action: Evolving innovative practice*. San Francisco, CA: Jossey-Bass.

Kurtz, L. (2004). Support and self-help groups. In C. Garvin, L. Gutierrez, and M. Galinsky (Eds.), *Handbook of Social Work Groups* (pp. 139-159). New York: Guilford Press.

LeDoux, J. (1998). Fear and the brain: Where have we been, and where are we going? *Biological Psychology*, 44(12): 1223-1238.

Lefcourt, H. and Davidson-Katz, K. (1991). Locus of control and health. In C.R. Snyder and D.R. Forsyth (Eds.), *Handbook of Social and Clinical Psychology: The Health Perspective* (pp. 246-266). New York: Pergamon Press.

Leiberman, M., Yalom, I., and Miles, M., (1972). Impact on participants. In Solomon and Berzon (Eds.), *New Perspectiveson Encounter Groups*, (pp. 119-170). San Francisco: Jossey-Bass, Inc.

Lesperance, F., Frasure-Smith, N., and Talajic, M. (1996). Major depression before and after myocardial infarction: Its nature and consequence. *Psychosomatic Medicine*, 58(2): 99-110.

Leszcz, M., Yalom, I., and Norden, M. (1985). The value of inpatient group psychotherapy and therapeutic process: Patients perceptions. *International Journal of Group Psychotherapy*, 35: 262-268.

Levenson, J. and Olbrisch, M. (1993). Psychosocial evaluation of organ transplant candidates: A comparative survey of process, criteria, and outcomes in heart, liver, and kidney transplantation. *Psychosomatics*, 34: 314-323.

Lewis, J., Rosen, R., and Goldstein, I. (2005). Erectile dysfunction. *Nursing*, 35(2): 64-68.

Lindsay, P., Sherrard, H., Bickerton, L., Doucette, P., Harkness, C., and Mortin, J. (1997). Educational and support needs of patients and their families awaiting cardiac surgery. *Heart and Lung*, 26(6): 458-465.

Lubin, H., Loris, M., and Burk, J. (1998). Efficacy of pschoeducational group therapy in reducing symptoms of posttraumatic stress disorder among multiple traumatized women. *American Journal of Psychiatry*, 155(9): 1172-1177.

Lucas, C. and Ledgerwood, A. (2004). Illicit street drugs and vascular injury. In N. Rich, K. Mattox, and A. Hirschberg (Eds.), *Vascular Trauma*. (2nd ed.) (pp. 421-426). Philadelphia, PA: W.B. Saunders.

Lucas, C., Ledgerwood, A., and Kline, R. (2000). Alcohol and drugs. In K. Mattox, D. Feliciano, and E. Moore (Eds.), *Trauma*, (pp. 1059-1074). New York, NY: McGraw-Hill.

Ludwig, A. and Farrelly, F. (1967). The weapons of insanity. *American Journal of Psychotheraphy* 21(4): 737-747.

Manolio, T. (2004). U.S. trends in prevalence of low coronary risk: National Health and Nutrition Examination Surveys. *Circulation*, 109: 32.

Maxmen, J. (1978). An educative model for inpatient group therapy. *International Journal of Group Psychotherapy*, 34(3): 355-368.

Mayou, R. (2005). Are psychological skills necessary in treating all physical disorders. *Australian and New Zealand Journal of Psychiatry*, 39(9): 800-806.

McLennan, M., Anderson, G., and Pain, K. (1996). Rehabilitation learning needs: Patient and family perceptions. *Patient Educational Counseling*, 27(2): 191-199.

Mercola, J. (1997). Stress control lowers cardiac risks. *Journal of Cardiology*, 157: 2213-2223.

Mercola, J. (1998). Stress on the job leads to heart attack. *Journal of Cardiology*, 88: 382-388.

Mercola, J. (2000). Anger test may identify those at risk of heart attack. *Journal of Cardiology*, 5: 76-85.

Mercola, J. (2002). Stress management may help heart disease patients. *American Journal of Cardiology*, 89: 1-15.

Miller, W. and Rollnick, S. (1991). *Motivational interviewing: Preparing people to change addictive behaviors*. New York: Guilford Press.

Minuchin, S. (1974). *Families and family therapy*. Binghamton, NY: Haworth Press.

Mittleman, M., Lewis, R., Maclure, M., Sherwood, J., and Muller, J. (2001). Triggering myocardial infarction by marijuana. *Circulation*, 103: 2805-2809.

Monaham, D., Kohman, M. and Coleman, M. (1996). Open-heat surgery: Consequences for caregivers. *Journal of Gerontological Social Work*, 25(n3-4): 53-68. Binghamton, NY: Haworth Press.

Moore, R. and Garland, A. (2003). *Cognitive therapy for chronic and persistent depression.* New York: John Wiley & Sons, Ltd.

Mosca, L., Ferris, A., Fabunmi, R., and Robertson, R. (2004). American Heart Association. Tracking women's awareness of heart disease: an American Heart Association national study. *Circulation,* 109: 573-579.

Mosca, L., Jones, W., King, K., Ouyang, P., Redberg, R., and Hill, M. (2000). Awareness, perception, and knowledge of heart disease risk and prevention among women in the United States: American Heart Association Women's Heart Disease and Stroke Campaign Task Force. *Archives of Family Medicine,* 9: 506-515.

Myerburg, R., Kessler, K., and Castellanos, A. (1993). Sudden cardiac death: Epidemiology, transient risk, and intervention assessment. *Annals of Internal Medicine,* 119: 1187-1197.

Myers, J. (1995). Survey results confirm prior belief but contradict conventional wisdom. *CHASER News,* 2(1): 6-8.

Natarajan, S., Liao, Y., Cao, G., Lipsitz, S., and McGee, D. (2003). Sex differences in risk for coronary heart disease mortality associated with diabetes and established coronary heart disease. *Archives of Internal Medicine,* 163: 1735-1740.

National Advisory Mental Health Council (1993). Health care reform for Americans with severe mental illnesses. *American Journal of Psychiatry,* 150(10): 1447-1465.

National Center for Chronic Disease Prevention and Health Promotion (NCCDPHP) (2001). *Behavioral risk factor surveillance system (BRFSD).* Hayattsville, MD National Center for Chronic Disease Prevention Health Promotion, Centers for Disease Control, and Prevention.

National Center for Chronic Disease Prevention and Health Promotion (NCCDPHP) (2005). *Preventing heart disease and stroke addressing the nation's leading killers.* Atlanta, GA: Centers for Disease Control and PreventionNational Center for Health Statistics. (2004). *Vital Health Statistics,* 13(157).

National Heart, Lung, and Blood Institute (1999). *Cardiovascular disease statistics,* (pp. 51-76). Bethesda, MD: National Institutes of Health.

National Heart, Lung, and Blood Institute (2002). *Women's heart disease statistics. National Institutes of Health,* (pp. 1-2). Bethesda, MD: National Institutes of Health.

National Institute on Drug Abuse (NIDA) Research Monograph, Number 108. (1991). *Cardiovascular toxicity of cocaine: Underlying mechanisms.* Baltimore, MD: U.S. Department of Health and Human Services.

National Institute on Drug Abuse (2005). *Research report series—Cocaine abuse and addiction.* National Institutes of Health (NIH) and the Baltimore, MD: U.S. Department of Health and Human Services.

National Institute of Mental Health (1999). *Facts about generalized anxiety disorder.* Bethesda, MD: U.S. Department of Health and Human Services.

National Institute of Mental Health (2001). NIMH Research on Women's Mental Health: Highlights FY 1999-FY 2000. Available at: www.nimh.nih.gov/wmhc/highlights.cfm. Accessed Jan. 24, 2002.

National Institute of Mental Health (2002). *Depression and heart disease: A fact sheet that summarizes what heart disease patients need to know about depression.* Bethesda, MD: U.S. Department of Health and Human Services.

National Institute of Mental Health (2003). *Facts about generalized anxiety disorder.* Bethesda, MD: U.S. Department of Health and Human Services.

National Institute of Mental Health (2005). *Depression: What every woman should know.*Bethesda, MD: U.S. Department of Health and Human Services.

National Institute of Mental Health (2006). *Panic disorder, a real illness.* Bethesda, MD: U.S. Department of Health and Human Services.

National Medicaid Expenditure Panel Survey (1987). Washington, DC: Centers for Medicare and Medicaid.

Nemeroff, C., Musselman, D., and Evans, D. (1998). Depression and cardiac disease. *Depression and Anxiety,* 8(suppl 1): 71-79. Bethesda, MD: National Institutes of Health.

Newman, M., Blumenthal, J., and Mark, D. (2004). Fixing the heart: Must the brain pay the price? *Circulation,* 110: 3402-3403.

New York Academy of Medicine (American Psychosomatic Society) (2004). *Risk of developing future heart disease.* Available from: URL: http:/www.ryan.org/news/112qhtlm.

New York Heart Association (2002). *New York heart association classification for congestive heart failure.* New York, NY Chapter: American Heart Association.

Nichols, M. and Schwartz, R. (1998). *Family therapy: Concepts and methods*, (4th ed.). New York: Allyn & Bacon.

O'Grady, D. (1998). *No hard feelings: Managing anger and conflict in your work, family, and love life* (Book on tape). AudioQueue.

Olbrisch, M. and Levenson, J. (1991). Psychosocial evaluation of heart transplant candidates: An international survey of process, criteria, and outcomes. *The Journal of Heart and Lung Transplantationi,* 10: 948-955.

Papadopoulous, C. (1989). Sexual aspects of cardiovascular disease. *Sexual Medicine, Volume 10.* New York: Praeger Publishers.

Penninx, B., Beekman, A., Honig, A., Deeg, D., Schoevers, R., van Eijk, J., and van Tilburg, W. (2001). Depression and cardiac mortality: Results from a community-based longitudinal study. *Archives of General Psychiatry,* 58(3): 221-227.

Perlman, H. (1970). *Social casework: A problem-solving process.* Chicago: University of Chicago Press.

Plach, S. (2002). Anxiety in women with heart disease. *Psychiatric Times* XIX(3).

Plach, S. and Heidrich, S. (2002). Social role quality, physical health, and psychological well-being in women after heart surgery. *Research in Nursing & Health,* 25: 189-202.

Plass, K. (2002). Like a bunch of cattle: The patient's experience of the outpatient health care environment. In S.P. Thomas and H.R. Pollo (Eds.) *Listen to Patients: A Phenomenological Approach to Nursing research and Practice* (pp. 237-251). New York: Springer Publishing.

Pranzarone, G. (02/1978). *Personal communication: Thoughts of human sexuality.* Roanoke, College, Salem, VA.

Pratt, L., Ford, D., and Crum, R. (1996). Depression, psychotropic medication, and the risk of myocardial infarction: Prospective data from the Baltimore ECA follow-up. *Circulation*, 94(12): 3123-3129.

Prochaska, J. and DiClemente, C. (1992). The transtheoretical approach. In J. Norcross and M. Golfried (Eds.), *Handbook of Psychotherapy Integration* (pp. 300-334). New York: Basic Books.

Prochaska, J., Norcross, J., and DiClemente (1994). *Changing for good: A revolutionary six-stage program for overcoming bad habits and moving your life positively forward.* New York: Avon Books.

Psychosocial Aspects of Transplantation (2002). Organ transplantation: Concepts, issues, practice, and outcomes. *Organ Transplant*, Medscape: Section 5(9).

Pucci, A. (2005). Evidence-based counseling and psychotherapy. *National Association of Cognitive-Behavioral Therapists.* Weirton, WV http://www.nacbt.org/evidence-based-therapy.htm

Purk, J. (2004). Support groups: Why do people attend? *Rehabilitation Nursing*, 29(2): 62-67.

Reid, W. (1992). *Task strategies: An empirical approach to social work practice.* New York: Columbia University Press.

Reid, W. (1996). Task-centered social work. In F. Turner (Ed.). *Social Work Treatment*, (4th ed.) (pp. 617-640). New York: The Free Press.

Robinson, V. (1930). *A changing psychology of social casework.* Chapel Hill, NC: University of North Carolina Press.

Roffman, R. (2004). Psychoeducational groups. In C. Garvin, L. Gutierrez, and M. Galinsky, (Eds.), *Handbook of Social Work Groups* (pp. 160-175). New York: Guilford Press.

Rogers, J. (2000). Heart patients, stay calm—Stress and cardiovascular disease. *Psychology Today*, March. New York: Sussex Publishing, Inc.

Rogers, W., Canto, J., Lambrew, C., Tiefenbrunn, A., Kinkaid, B., Shoultz, D., and Frederick, P., Every, N. (2000). Temporal trends in the treatment of over 1.5 million patients with myocardial infarction in the US from 1990 through 1999: The National Registry of Myocardial Infarction 1, 2 and 3. *Journal of American College of Cardiologist*, 36: 2056-2063.

Rollins, J. (1987). Self-help groups for parents. *Pediatric Nursing*, 13: 403-409.

Rollnick, S. and Butler, C. (2003). *Rapid reference to compliance: Rapid reference series.* Oxford, UK: Churchill Livingstone.

Rollnick, S., Mason, P., and Butler, C. (1999). *Health behavior change: A guide for practitioners.* Oxford, UK: Churchill Livingstone.

Rosenstock, I. (1974). Historical origins of the health belief model. *Health Education Monographs*, 2(4): 1-4.

Rozanski, A., Blumenthal, A., and Kaplan, J. (1999). Impact of psychological factors on the pathogenesis of cardiovascular disease and implications for therapy. *Circulation*, 99: 2192-2117.

Rudisch, B. and Nemeroff, C. (2003). Epidemiology of comorbid coronary artery disease and depression. *Biological Psychiatry*, 54(3): 227-240.

Rutledge, T. and Hogan, B. (2002). A quantitative review of prospective evidence linking psychological factors with hypertension development. *Psychosomatic Medicine*, 64: 758-766.

Rutledge, T., Linden, W., and Paul, D. (2002). The reliability of cardiovascular reactivity: Effects of task-type & family history over a 3-year interval. *International Journal of Behavioral Medicine*, 8: 293-303.

Schwartz, E. and Rodriguez, J. (2005). Sex and the heart. *International Journal of Impotence Research*, 17: S4-S6.

Schwartzben, S. (1992). Social work with multi-family groups: A partnership model for long term care settings. *Social Work in Health Care*, 18(1): 23-38.

Sexton, T. and Alexander, J. (1999). *Functional Family Therapy: Principles of Clinical Intervention.* Henderson, NV: RCH Enterprises.

Sexton, T. and Alexander, J. (2000). Functional family therapy. *Juvenile Justice Bulletin.* Washington, DC: U.S. Department of Justice.

Shulman, L. (1983). The professional connection with self-help groups in health care settings. *Social Work in Health Care*, 8(4): 69-77.

Sipski, M. and Alexander, C. (1997). *Sexual function in people with disability and chronic illness: A health professional's guide.* Gaithersburg, MD: Aspen.

Skinner, B. (1950). Are theories of learning necessary? *Psychological Review*, 57(4): 193-216.

Sorensent, C., Friis-Hasche, E., Haghfelt, T., and Beck, P. (2005). Postmyocardial infarction mortality in relation to depression: A. systematic critical review. *Psychotherapy and Psychosomatcs*, 74(2): 69-80.

Starak, Y. (1982). Co-leadership: A new look at sharing group work. *Social Work with Groups*, 4(3/4): 145-157.

Strong Heart Study Data Book (2001). *NHLBI.* Washington, DC: National Institutes Health.

Stull, D., Starling, R., Hass, G., and Young, J. (1999). Becoming a patient with heart failure. *Heart and Lung*, 28(4): 284-292.

Substance Abuse and Mental Health Services Administration (SAMHA) (2004). *Results from the 2003 national survey on drug use and health: National findings.* NSDUH Series H-25. DHHS Pub. No. (SMA) 04-3964. Rockville, MD: DHHS.

Suszycki, L. (1986). Social work groups on a heart transplant program. *Journal of Heart Transplant*, 5(2): 166-170.

Tata, L. (2005). Heart attack risks linked to depression not antidepressants. *Heart*, 91: 465-471.

Tavris, C. (1982). *Anger: The misunderstood emotion.* New York: Simon & Schuster.

Thomas, S. (1989). Gender differences in anger expression: Health implications. *Research in Nursing and Health*, 12: 389-398.

Thomas, S. and Donnellan, M. (1993). Stress, role responsibilities, social support, and anger. In S.P. Thomas (Ed.), *Women and Anger* (pp. 112-128). New York: Springer.

Thomas, S., Smucker, C., and Droppleman, P. (1998). It hurts most around the heart: A phenomenological exploration of women's anger. *Journal of Advanced Nursing*, 28(2): 311-322.

Tiba, A. and Szentagotai, A. (2005). Positive emotions and irrational beliefs: Dysfunctional positive emotions in healthy individuals. *Aurora; Journal of Cognitive & Behavioral Psychotherapies*, 5(1): 53-72.

Tice, D. and Baumeister, R. (1993). Controlling anger: Self-induced emotion change. In D.M. Wegner and J. Pennebaker (Eds.), *Handbook of Mental Control* (pp. 393-409). Englewood Cliffs, NJ: Prentice Hall.

Toseland, R., Jones, L., and Gellis, Z. Group dynamics. (2004). In C. Garvin, L. Gutierrez, and M. Galinsky (Eds.), *Handbook of Social Work Groups* (pp. 13-31). New York: Guilford Press.

Tsaih, S., Korrick, S., Schwartz, J., Amarasiriwardena, C., Aro, A., Sparrow, D., and Hu, H. (2004). Lead, diabetes, hypertension, and renal function: The normative aging study. *Environmental Health Perspectives*, 112(11): 1178-1182.

Turner, J. and Jaco, R. (1996). Problem-solving theory and social work treatment. In F. Turner (Ed.), *Social Work Treatment*, (4th ed.) (pp. 503-522). New York: The Free Press.

United Network for Organ Sharing (UNOS) (2005). *United States heart transplant statistics*. United Network for Organ Sharing. Washington, DC: U.S. Department of Health and Human Services (HHS) and the Health Resources and Services Administration (HRSA).

Van Andel, P., Erdman, R., Karsdorp, P., Apples, A., and Trijsburg, R. (2003). Group cohesion and working alliance: Prediction of treatment outcome in cardiac patients receiving cognitive behavioral group psychotherapy. *Psychotherapy and Psychosomatics*, 72(3): 141-149.

Van Peski-Oosterbann, A., Spinhoven, P., Van der Does, A., Bruschke, A., and Rooijmans, H. (1999). Cognitive change following cognitive behavioral therapy for non-cardiac chest pain. *Psychotherapy and Psychosomatics*, 68: 214-220.

Waller J. (1972). Nonhighway injury fatalities. I. The roles of alcohol and problem drinking, drugs and medical impairment. *Journal of Chronic Diseases*, 25: 33-45.

Walter, P., Mohan, R., and Dahan-Mizrahl, S. (1992). Quality of life after open heart surgery. *Quality of Life Research*, 1(1): 77-83.

Watkins, L. and Blumenthal, J. (1999). Worried to death? (Correspondence). *Circulation*, 100: 1250-1252.

Weinert, C. (2005). Epidemiology and treatment of psychiatric conditions that develop after critical illness. *Current Opinion on Critical Care*, 11(4): 376-380.

West, S., Vinikoor, L., and Zolnoun, D. (2004). A systematic review of the literature on female sexual dysfunction prevalence and predictors. *The Annual Review of Sex Research*, Volume 15. Washington, DC: The Society for the Scientific Study of Sexuality.

Whitehill, D. (2005).Viagra, Levitra, and Cialis: what's the difference? *South Dakota Journal of Medicine*, 58(4): 129-130.

Williams, J., Paton, C., Siegler, I., Eigenbrodt, M., Nieto, F., and Tyroler, H. (2000). Anger proneness predicts coronary heart disease risk: Prospective analysis from the Atherosclerosis Risk in Communities (ARIC) Study. *Circulation*, 101: 2034-2039.

Winkelmayer, C. (2005). Habitual caffeine intake and the risk of hypertension in women. *The Journal of American Medical Association*, 294: 2330-2335.

Woods, M. and Robinson, H. (1996). Psychosocial theory and social work treatment. In F. Turner (Ed.), *Social Work Treatment*, (4th ed.) (pp. 555-580). New York: The Free Press.

Yalom, I. (1980). *Existential psychotherapy.* New York: Basic Books.

Yalom, I. (1995) *Theory and practice of group psychotherapy.* (4th ed.). New York: Basic Books.

Young, J. (2003). *Cognitive therapy for personality disorders: A schema-focused approach (practitioner's resource series).* New York: Guilford Press.

Young, J., Weishaar, M., and Klosko, J. (1999). *Schema therapy: A practitioner's guide.* New York: Guilford Press.

Zheng, Z., Croft, J., Giles, W., and Mensah, G. (2001). Sudden cardiac death in the United States, 1989 to 1998. *Circulation,* 104: 2158-2163.

Ziegeistein, R., Fauerbach, J., and Stevens, S. (2000). Patients with depression are less likely to follow recommendation to reduce cardiac risk during recovery from a myocardial infarction. *Archives of Internal Medicine,* 160(12): 1818-1823.

Index

Abandonment, as cognitive schema, 44
Acarbose, 90-91
Acceptance
  of others, 154
  as response to grief, 143-144
Accidents
  alcohol use-related, 161
  as mortality cause, 5
Acetazolamide, effect on sexual
    function, 177
Activities, unproductive, 138
Adherence, with treatment. *See*
    Compliance, with treatment
Adjustment difficulties, cognitive-
    behavioral group therapy for,
    39
Adrenaline, 16
African Americans, cardiovascular
    disease in, 88
  heart failure, 99
  as mortality cause, 4, 6
  risk factors for, 8
  treatment of, 9-10
African-American women,
    cardiovascular disease risk in,
    7, 9
Aggression, anger-related, 143, 144
Aggressive personality trait, 145
Agreements/contracts, in social group
    work, 32-33
Alcohol use
  contraindication in heart failure
    patients, 102
  effect on sexual function, 176
  excessive, 62, 75, 160-161
  limited, 89
  moderate, 93, 159, 161
  positive cardiovascular effects of,
    93, 161-162
Allergies, as stress cause, 133

Alpha methyldopa, effect on sexual
    function, 177
American College of
    Cardiology/American Heart
    Association, heart failure
    classification system of, 98-99
American Group Psychotherapy
    Association, 29
American Health Association, 172
American Heart Association, 18, 85,
    87, 89, 97, 161-162
American Indians
  cardiovascular disease incidence in,
    5
  cardiovascular disease-related
    mortality in, 4, 6
  heart attack incidence among, 5
American Medical Association, 159,
    161-162
American Psychiatric Association, 19,
    129
Amiodipine, 20
Amitryptyline, effect on sexual
    function, 177
Amphetamines, 159
Anger, 22-25, 37
  adverse health effects of, 143,
    144-145
  as cardiovascular disease cause,
    19-20, 22-25, 39, 40-41, 92
  cognitive-behavioral group therapy
    for, 39, 40-41
  as coronary heart disease risk factor,
    23-24
  definition of, 144
  as depression risk factor, 22-23, 40
  effect on interpersonal relationships,
    153-154
  as externalized depression, 22-23
  as hypertension risk factor, 92